ADVANCE PRAISE FOR

Outwitting Headaches

"Mark Wiley pulls no punches in empowering you to stop your head-aches with a thorough integrative, natural, mind body approach. His writing skills make for an enjoyable ride to pain-free living. I believe this program will do more for everyone than just cure headaches—it is a healing, healthy, preventative lifestyle for us all! Read it, Do it, and Enjoy life again."

—**Gary D. Sandman**
Founder, Individual Health Solutions
Editor-in-Chief, HealUSA.net

"Those chronic headache victims who search for relief from Western medicine alone reach a dead end pretty quickly. That's where Dr. Mark Wiley comes in. Combining the latest Western medical research with proven Eastern medical techniques, he presents a fully integrated ap-proach to eliminating headaches forever. If you suffer from this kind of pain, your path to recovery begins with this book."

—**Brian Saint-Paul**
Editor, *CRISIS* Magazine

"Chronic pain is a major problem in our modern society. Stress, poor diet, lack of sleep, improper breathing, dehydration, toxins, chemicals . . . all lead to congestion and block the innate energy within us that makes us move, keeps us healthy. Chronic headache sufferers can find the relief they're looking for in the pages of this fine book. In *Outwitting Headaches*, Dr. Wiley clearly and succinctly points the way; it's up to you to follow it."

—The Association of Clinical Qigong

"In my years of clinical practice, I have found Dr. Wiley's self-help headache program to be the best in terms of headache treatment. I use it with great success in my own clinic and recommend his book, *Outwitting Headaches*, to all people—headache sufferers and health care professionals alike."

—Alan Orr
Acupuncturist (London, England)

"With the growing epidemic of headaches in the world from stress, over-the-counter medication abuses, prescription drugs, poor diet, and traumas of everyday life, this book is essential for the individual who desires to be free of the debilitating effects of headaches. Dr. Wiley's compelling story and integrated self-directed program will give any headache sufferer the belief: "If he can do it, so can I!""

—Dr. Brett D. Cardonick
Cardonick Chiropractic (Philadelphia, PA)

"History has shown that while doctors and healers the world over are able to ease the symptoms of headache, none can promise a cure. Dr. Wiley's personal suffering and tireless research into the subject clearly shows that the only way to rid ourselves of them is through what he calls a *self-directed and integrated mind-body approach*. *Outwitting Headaches* clearly establishes the need for such a program, and the results will amaze you. If you're in search of truly lasting headache relief, this book is a must!"

—Robert Chu, L.Ac., QME
Oasis Vitality Center (Los Angeles, CA)

Outwitting Headaches

Outwitting Headaches

The Eight-Part Program for Total and Lasting Headache Relief

Mark V. Wiley, OMD.

THE LYONS PRESS
Guilford, Connecticut

An imprint of The Globe Pequot Press

The Lyons Press is an imprint of The Globe Pequot Press

10 9 8 7 6 5 4 3 2 1

Printed in the United States of America

Library of Congress Cataloging-in-Publication Data

.Wiley, Mark V.
  Outwitting headaches : the eight-part program for total and lasting headache relief / Mark V. Wiley.
      p. cm.
  Includes bibliographical references and index.
  ISBN 1-59228-264-4 (trade paper)
  1. Headache--Popular works. I. Title.
RC392.W539 2004
616.8'491--dc22

                                                      2004014241

Dedication

I lovingly dedicate this book to my parents, Drs. William and Mary Wiley, and to my sister, Mary Armstrong. For nearly three decades, they suffered my headaches alongside me and, despite my daily pain and irritability, showed me nothing but understanding, patience, and love.

Tong ze be tong; Bu tong ze tong.
If there is free flow, there is no pain;
If there is pain, there is no free flow.
　　　　—Axiom of Chinese Medicine

Contents

Foreword

It is my pleasure to write this foreword for Mark V. Wiley, O.M.D., a friend and a skilled healer. As a chronic sufferer of headaches, he took it upon himself to search far and wide for methods and disciplines to overcome his torment and pain. Actually, his personal journey to pain relief is most compelling.

Mark spent years in a seemingly endless search for a lasting cure for his headache pain. He met pain specialists in many fields of medicine here in the United States, and then he located and visited traditional healers in a half-dozen Asian countries. Sometimes the treatments worked, and sometimes they didn't. But that didn't deter him; he kept on searching. After he saw what worked for him and at what times and under what circumstances, he was able to begin an analysis of *why* some of the treatment results were more profound and longer-lasting than others.

When Mark put all of this information together, he came to realize that one healing modality worked sometimes while others worked at other times (or not at all). It depended on the root cause of the headache, its location in the head, and how many factors contributed to its duration. It became apparent to him that a majority of the chronic headaches that plagued him (and millions of other people) could be averted completely with the right kind of global lifestyle changes. In other words, if you do not allow those things that *trigger* a headache to take hold in the body, *the headache will not come.* It's that simple!

In my own busy clinic, I often see patients suffering from debilitating headaches, where their quality of life is diminished and they are unable to properly do their work, study, or take care of family. Even simple tasks become a chore when there is a severe headache. And I can't begin to tell you how many patients I see who suffer headaches and continue to take prescription and over-the-counter medications—even though there is no lasting relief of pain. And it is these very medications that are used to treat the headache pain that are harming their livers or interrupting their days with frequent bouts of diarrhea, muscle aches, lack of clarity, and other troublesome side effects. Often, the treatment can be worse than the disease!

At the Oasis Vitality Center in Pasadena, California, I employ a combination of acupuncture, herbal therapy, meditation/qigong, dietary changes, nutritional counseling, and stress relief techniques to bring about a therapeutic result. And while the results are satisfactory, the headaches sometimes appear again—sometimes sooner than later. Over the years, many of my patients have remarked that at times when their schedules are hectic, when work extends into overtime hours, or when they must take care of their small children, they wished they had a method of immediate headache relief or a means of preventing headaches altogether. Unfortunately, I had nothing to recommend to them—until now.

Outwitting Headaches clearly delineates methods for treating all types of headaches, whether you suffer from chronic mixed headaches; migraine and cluster headaches; allergy, sensitivity, and diet-induced headaches; oxygen and sleep deprivation headaches; or stress, tension-type, or structural headaches. There are eight simple aspects to the program and there is also an emergency intervention to cut off a headache during its attack. Each aspect of the program is based on sound scientific studies, and the methods espoused therein come from a wide range of healing modalities. Best of all, the program depends only on the desire of the individual sufferer to want to do it. It is for these reasons that I believe *Outwitting Headaches* is a milestone in self-help books.

History has shown that while doctors and healers the world over are able to ease the symptoms of headaches, none can promise a cure. Mark Wiley's personal suffering and tireless research into the subject clearly shows that the only way to rid yourself of them is through what he calls a "self-directed and integrated mind/body approach." *Outwitting Headaches* clearly establishes the need for such a program, and the results will amaze you.

Every person would do well to have a copy of this book on his or her shelf, and I highly recommend it to other physicians to help their patients who suffer from debilitating headaches. Executives, athletes, and small business owners can also find relief here in times of great stress. *Outwitting Headaches* truly is a self-directed and integrated mind/body approach to dealing with headaches. If you're in search of truly lasting headache relief, this book is a must!

Robert Chu, L.Ac., Ph.D.
Director of Oriental Medicine
Oasis Vitality Center
Pasadena, CA

Acknowledgments

No work is ever conceived or produced in a vacuum, and this present work is no exception. Of course, the genesis of my research into a cure for headaches goes back to my childhood suffering. I really must credit the caring and open-mindedness of my father (an osteopath) and my mother (a psychologist), who took me from specialist to specialist in search of relief. It was these visits to hospitals and specialists' offices, coupled with books on Asian philosophy and acupuncture on my parents' bookshelves while I was a child, that gave me the initial interest in Oriental and so-called alternative medicine.

An acknowledgment needs to be given to those trail-blazing American doctors who saw the effectiveness and need for alternative methods of achieving health and healing. It is these individuals who became the first writers on holistic and traditional healing in the United States, who offered much of the Western world their first, and sometimes only, glimpses into methods of healing "foreign" to their own soil. To the following doctors, whose works have been my inspiration, I offer my sincere gratitude and respect: Andrew Weil, M.D.; Herbert Benson, M.D.; Michael Maliszewski, Ph.D.; Ted Kaptchuk, O.M.D.; and David Eisenberg, M.D.

Of the hundreds of traditional healers I had the opportunity to meet, interview, learn from, and entrust my own health to, I would especially like to acknowledge the following healers for offering me so much time, knowledge, and support in my journey as a researcher, writer, and healer: Master FaXiang Hou; Robert Chu, L.Ac., Ph.D.; Ong Kok Seng, O.M.D.; Gangsham Gyanagarker, Ph.D.; Master Jose Mena; Master Cheong Cheng Leong; Master Tan Hun Poy; Guru M. Subramaniam; Master Sam Tendencia; Gat Puno Abun Baet; Manghi-hilot Rico Dalay; Master David Chan; Rene Navarro, L.Ac.; Tom Bisio, L.Ac.; and Master Alan Orr.

At this point I must also offer my thanks to Reynalso S. Galang for accompanying me on my first trip to Manila and introducing me to Alexander Co, who so unselfishly arranged for me to meet so many traditional healers in the Philippines and Taiwan. To Ron Beaubien and Alexander Kask for assisting my research in Japan. To Hunter Armstrong and S. Karunakaran for their assistance with my research in Malaysia. Again to Michael Maliszewski, Ph.D., of Harvard Medical School, for a tremendous overall exposure to the alternative sides of mind/body healing. To Christoph Amberger, M.A., publisher of *Taipan,* for giving me a wonderful opportunity to launch a health publication from the ground up, which led to my meeting Gary Sandman and the opportunity to write for HealUSA.net. To Herb Borkland, for his endless inspiration and support. And to George Donahue, my forgiving and sincere editor, for believing in this project and, with his associates at The Lyons Press, bringing it to publication.

Of course, if not for the love and strength I derive from my wife, Janet, and son, Alexander, I would not be living the life of my dreams.

Outwitting Headaches

Introduction

Do you get headaches? How often, how bad? The reason I ask is my male vanity. I keep telling myself that I'm the King of Pain. My migraines? Every day for twenty-seven years. Cute ones, too. For instance, one fall day, as I walked along Philadelphia's Schuylkill River, positive thoughts of the future filled my mind. Life was good. Twenty seconds later, I wanted to die.

It struck from behind, like a truck slamming into a wall. Pain seared through my head as effortlessly as a chainsaw glides through balsa wood. My head felt like it was at once being crushed from the outside and pushed apart from the inside. At the same time, it felt like someone was jamming a screwdriver into my right eye, while a rock was being wedged under the base of my skull. Shivers, cold sweats, and shaky knees forced me to drop in pain, gasp for air.

To deaden the pain, I began scraping my forehead across the ground and then along the cool stone wall. Lunch came back up on me as violently as a dam suddenly broken by the force of a raging flood. Deep, dark spots and burning tears obstructed my vision as I begged for death. But I was intimate with this pain, and I knew very well that neither death nor God would come to my rescue.

Yet this was only an average attack—not even close to being one of the worst. It was just another in the lifelong series of daily migraine, cluster, tension, toxic, and rebound headaches I experienced for nearly three decades. And this, despite having seen some of the best-trained physicians of Western medicine and taking an average of fourteen capsules of various medications a day. Every day.

The constant, uncontrollable suffering was destroying me. I couldn't exercise on a regular basis because of severe headaches caused by jumping, running, and lifting. This was particularly demoralizing as I was a professional martial artist. In college, I had to do extracurricular work to make up for missed classes and exams as a result of being bedridden. I knew that if the headaches kept recurring on this schedule for much longer I would, in the immortal words of Ed Grimly, "Go mental!"

You see, I began life two-and-a-half months premature, weighing in at only one pound, nine ounces. My first four months were spent in the hospital. I had below-average bone development, and I experienced breathing difficulties and infantile spasms now believed to have been deep seizures. Doctors now think that all this resulted in the chronic musculoskeletal pain and headaches that dogged me since childhood (or perhaps since birth).

My parents selflessly spent a tremendous amount of time and money trying to cure these pains the Western way. To no avail. By the time I was thirteen, I was experiencing what are known as rebound headaches—that is, additional headaches caused by the body's reaction to the combination and sheer amount of prescription and over-the-counter medications in my system. At different times I was prescribed beta blockers and a calcium channel blocker; at one point I was even taking a combination of two Midrin, two Fioricet, and two Excedrin at one swallow—several times a day! This didn't always relieve the pain, nor did it keep it from recurring. When the prescription capsules were unable to do their job, and my headache pain was severe beyond description, I would be taken to the emergency room where both Demoral and Sumatriptan intravenously entered into my system, along with an antivomiting drug. Even with this, it would often take an additional 4 hours for the pain to dissipate. In short, while Western methods did treat the symptoms of the headache (i.e., pain, aura, cold sweats, nausea), they did my headache pain no lasting good and my body some short-term harm.

In 1982, my father introduced me to his chiropractor, Dr. John Sears, thus beginning my journey in alternative health and wellness. I spent the better part of the 1990s traveling around the world to meet with traditional healers in the United States, England, Japan, Taiwan, Malaysia, Singapore, and the Philippines. I sought out those rumored Eastern geniuses of so-called "alternative" and "holistic" medicine whose waiting rooms their patients reached by climbing mountains or hacking through jungles. Acupuncturists in Japan, qigong masters in Taiwan, bone setters in Malaysia, faith healers in the Philippines . . . Been there, done that.

To my dismay, I found that while their methods of diagnosis and treatment are diametrically opposed to and far less invasive than the Western model, their treatments actually offered no greater long-term relief from my chronic headaches. I knew that there was something natural and powerful in what these traditional methods offered, but I felt a burning need to know exactly why the short-term successes did not turn into long-term results.

Over a twelve-year period of apprenticeship, intense study, and clinical training in Asia, the United States, and the United Kingdom, I earned a doctorate in Oriental medicine and master-level certificates in clinical and orthopedic qigong, tuina bodywork and manipulation therapy, Chinese herbal medicine and diet therapy, and other related fields.

I came to understand the diagnostic and treatment principles of the Asian systems of healing and believed in them wholeheartedly. But still the headaches came.

Then it happened: One morning I just woke up and decided that I had had enough. I decided to take my health and well-being into my own hands, rather than expecting someone else to take care of them for me. I read every book and journal study I could find on headache etiology and treatment. I met with leading experts in Western pain management and Eastern alternative therapies to discuss the topic and my condition and observations. It wasn't until I stepped back from the forest that I saw the trees, each one of them individually, for the first time. It was then that I began to really understand the variety of factors causing the headaches, and the answer to eliminating the "triggers" from my life and, by extension, the headaches themselves.

In fact, I was so amazed with the results of my *self-directed, self-cure program* that I immediately started telling my friends and co-workers about it. I was like an evangelist, praising the powers of an *integrated mind/body approach* to curing headaches. Many were skeptical. After all, they argued, if such a simplistic approach could work, wouldn't the greatest minds in medical science be professing it? I reasoned that perhaps the mainstream medical establishment did know the answer, but since my approach dismissed the need for Western pharmaceuticals they had no interest in promoting such a program.

But this view was not completely fair. Actually, there are a growing number of mainstream physicians who do advocate complementary and alternative medicine as an adjunct to their biomed approach. I researched their programs, books, and studies and found much technical evidence supporting the different parts of my headache program. To my amazement, though, while many medical researchers and health care providers advocated one or another aspect of my program as a powerful tool when *combined with* Western medicine, none of them saw the entire scope of the problem for what it is, and none of them connected all the components.

Bottom line? After nearly thirty years of skull-melting, eye-blinding headache pain, I finally reached the top of the mountain, put all the wisdom together—conventional or not—and I am here to tell you, I killed the monsters forever. And now I want to tell you how you can kill them, too, and get on with a life worth living.

It took several years to work out the details and sequence of the program, but in the end it was a *self-directed integrated mind/body approach* that removed these monsters from my life. Once I was able to control the headaches, the headaches were never again able to control me.

Given the right information and the proper motivation, you can take back control of your life by taking a proactive role in your own state of health and wellness, rather than a passive one where you are at the mercy of overworked, disinterested physicians who have no real stake in whether or not your condition improves or is removed. My own personal journey took twenty-seven years of trying and failing until I was so fed up by the return of the headaches that I dug a trench, settled in, and waged war on my chronic pain. You can too, and the following chapters will explain the whys and hows of outwitting headaches in language you can understand: types and causes of headaches, methods of treatment, specific things you can do to keep them from recurring, and what to do if they do come back.

To come to the point where you are psychologically ready to stop playing the role of victim to the headache and servant to the physician/healer takes great courage and discipline. I am confident that you have what it takes to outwit your headaches and take back control of your life. So do it. Do it now, without another moment's delay. I promise that your life will change in innumerable ways with the coming of lasting pain relief. Do it now, because no one except you gives a damn about the quality of *your* life. This book will show you the way. All you have to do is make and keep a personal promise and commitment to yourself that you will see it through to the end. It's your choice.

What's it going to be?

Chapter One

AN INTEGRATED
MIND/BODY APPROACH

The near future of prescription headache medication holds the promise of mind-boggling progress. The amount of research and development done by pharmaceutical, med-tech, and bio-tech companies that is being conducted today is staggering. And once research and development has been concluded and FDA trials have been passed, we're looking at a plethora of medical miracles heading our way.

There's just one problem: Medical progress comes at a price. It will never be cheap to treat chronic illnesses the high-tech way. In fact, medication for certain disorders can be so expensive that even the most generous HMO or health insurer will cut off the sufferer after a year or two.

The American health care system will always be bogged down by the high costs of pharmaceuticals, extended hospital stays, and sky-high insurance costs—and no amount of politicking will make the costs go away. It's the chronically ill who incur the lion's share of these costs over a long period of time. In many cases, that care can relieve and treat symptoms, but it often cannot provide a cure or put a final end to the pain or illness.

It's truly amazing that despite great advances in medical science, an astonishing twenty-six million Americans are suffering migraine headaches as part of their daily lives—70 percent of them women.[1] They accept them as inevitable and swallow prescription drugs as a matter of habit, just as they brush their teeth without giving the action a second thought. But chronic headaches take their toll, not only on the body's ability to maintain a state of homeostasis or wellness, but on the ability to think logically, see clearly, and feel and act appropriately. The impact all this has on one's quality of life is shattering: jobs lost, relationships ruined, motivation diminished, and happiness disintegrated.

How Headaches Become Chronic

Through common methods of socialization such as television, print media, and the general advice of physicians, our habitual response to headaches is to swallow over-the-counter analgesics and anti-inflammatories or prescription drugs. Time has undeniably shown that these do not provide us with long-term headache relief. In fact, while pain-relieving drugs are mainstays of many chronic-headache management programs, their long-term use adversely affects the digestive tract, the liver, and the kidneys through toxic buildup. This, of course, leads to the taking of more and more over-the-counter analgesics, which leads to more rebound headaches, which leads to taking stronger prescription medications, and so on in a vicious circle until the pain has gone from arising once in a while to being a chronic problem. And this makes the headache problem not only worse, but more difficult to treat and eventually eliminate.

In 1996 the journal *Health & Social Work* reported that seventy-seven million Americans suffer from chronic pain annually.[2] In 2002

The American Occupational Therapy Association (AOTA), reported that more than 130 million Americans suffer from chronic pain today. The AOTA further reports that "pain accounts for one-fourth of all sick days taken by full-time workers, costing the economy fifty billion lost workdays and $3 billion in lost wages."[3]

As if that weren't enough, chronic pain can decrease a person's strength, coordination, and independence. It also causes severe stress and can lead to depression. Chronic pain sufferers miss an average of four workdays per year and also shell out some of the $4 billion spent each year on over-the-counter pain relievers. Conversely, OnHealth.com reports that many pain clinics across the country are now advocating that the first step in many cases is to taper patients off their dependence on painkillers.[4]

The Western approach to health and healing still sees a Cartesian split between mind, body, and spirit. Conversely, the interconnection and interdependence of mind/body/spirit pervades the everyday life of traditional cultures the world over. In China, for example, they have been using a medical system which employs the high-tech lifesaving Western modes of surgeries and pharmaceuticals concurrently with the use of acupuncture, special diets, herbal remedies, and the practice of energy-building exercises known as qigong.

Some Alternatives

If you live in the United States and watch network television, you may have noticed that not a week goes by without the maternal triumvirate of Diane Sawyer, Barbara Walters, and Jane Pauley serving up warmed-over reruns of investigative reports on medical breakthroughs, alternative cures, and dietary supplements.

Undeniably, there's an increasing interest in alternative medicine these days. According to a national phone survey conducted by David Eisenberg, M.D., of Beth Israel Deaconess Medical Center in Boston, four out of every ten Americans use some kind of alternative medical treatment. Relaxation therapy, herbs, massage, and chiropractic care are among the most popular.[5] Accordingly, Americans are now spending millions of dollars of out-of-pocket money on alternative therapies each year. Nationwide, the alternative medicine and nutritional supplements industry is raking in close to a billion dollars annually.

In 1997 and 1998, Landmark Healthcare, Inc., commissioned studies regarding the public's and HMOs' perception of alternative health. The study found that 74 percent of people surveyed currently use alternative care along with traditional care. Sixty-seven percent said that they chose their HMO because it offered alternative care options, and 45 percent responded that they were willing to pay more for such plans. These studies also found that 67 percent of HMOs do offer at least one type of alternative care therapy, and that an additional 36 percent were most likely to cover acupuncture in the next two to three years. [6, 7]

Looking to alternative therapies for the curing of ailments or prevention thereof is nothing new. In fact, the 1970s saw a mass quantity of studies on the effects of placebos, self-hypnosis, biofeedback, fad diets, psychotropic drugs, and other alternative therapies from acupuncture to meditation, chiropractic to shamanism, and faith healing to psychic surgery.

Paavo Airola, Ph.D., wrote more than a dozen books on the subject during that decade, including *How To Get Well*. Originally published in 1974, by 1980 this book was reprinted no less than eighteen times, becoming a national bestseller. This was quite a feat at a time when Western pharmaceuticals and invasive surgery were center stage. Herbert

Benson, M.D., wrote *The Relaxation Response* in 1975, and in 1979, he followed it with *The Mind/Body Effect*. In these two books, he uncovered, discussed, and analyzed the mind/body connection in healing. Also published in 1979 was Norman Cousins's *Anatomy of an Illness as Perceived by the Patient*, published by Norton & Co., an analysis of how one man proved the mind can cure the body. This concise book went through a phenomenal thirteen printings before that year's end, only to be serialized in five magazines in 1980. It was then reprinted by Bantam in 1981, going on to spend an amazing forty weeks on the *New York Times* bestseller list.

In 1983, Andrew Weil, M.D., published his first book on alternative therapies. Simply titled *Health and Healing*, this book gave Americans their first well-rounded definition of health and an unbiased and well-researched presentation of nearly a dozen alternative therapies, from chiropractic to faith healing. It became an instant national bestseller, spawning greater nationwide acceptance of such healing modalities and a line of additional books by the author, including the bestseller *Spontaneous Healing*, again drawing the connection between the mind and body and their joined effects on curing illnesses.

The end of the '80s saw Deepak Chopra, M.D.'s *Quantum Healing*, which explored and offered new insights into the frontiers of mind/body medicine. Both this book and his 1993 work, *Timeless Body/Ageless Mind*, focused on the connection between biology, spirituality, and India's ayurvedic healing philosophies—and they became national bestsellers.

Bill Moyers's ground-breaking television documentary–turned–book, *Healing and the Mind*, became an instant national bestseller. This study focused on a cross-cultural and multidisciplinary approach to the connection of mind and body in health, healing, and wellness.

Along with the rest of the American population, headache sufferers are disenchanted with mainstream medical treatments for their chronic conditions and are turning instead to alternative therapies for answers on a regular basis. In fact, much to the chagrin of the entrenched medical establishment, the *Journal of the American Medical Association* (*JAMA*) reported that between 1990 and 1997 Americans had made 629 million visits to naturopaths, chiropractors, massage therapists, and other unconventional practitioners. This is double the amount of visits patients paid that same year to their primary care physicians! What's more, they spent $21.2 billion on those services—roughly $12 billion of which was their own hard-earned cash. That yearly out-of-pocket amount climbs to $27 billion when you throw in herbs, vitamins, and other over-the-counter health supplements.[7] The study attributes this substantial rise to "an increase in the proportion of the population seeking alternative therapies, rather than increased visits per patient."[8]

In 1998 another survey in *JAMA* offered a reason for this, reporting that the population was doing so "largely because they find these health care alternatives to be more congruent with their own values, beliefs, and philosophical orientations toward health and life."[9]

It is apparent that over the past thirty years alternative therapies have been lodging themselves more deeply into the American consciousness, becoming a permanent part of our collective psyche. It is no wonder, then, that in this new millennium an integrative mind/body approach to health is being seriously considered by Western medical practitioners as an adjunct to their practices. This, of course, begs the question of why, with the development of stronger drugs and the mainstream acceptance of alternative therapies, there are still a whopping forty-one million Americans suffering headaches annually?[10]

The Fundamental Problems

While I believe that it is better to have your pain temporarily removed by acupuncture and natural herbal remedies than with toxic biomedical drugs, these healing modalities often offer the same lackluster results as Western medicine: the temporary relief of pain and symptoms and not the prevention of the headaches themselves.

There are essentially two fundamental problems with modern biomedicine and traditional healing approaches. The headache sufferer is dependent on (1) the skills of the "healer" and (2) the strength of the "mechanism" (be it prescription drugs, acupuncture, or faith healing) to mask or lessen the symptoms of the pain and ailment. And a healer-dependent program will never put an end to headaches because it is predicated on managing symptoms.

Physicians view headaches as a puzzle to solve or a pathology to treat, and they take their time bothering with case histories and trying different medications and combinations until, years later, you are no better off than when you made the initial visits to their offices. In reality, it is highly likely that you may be worse off, since your body has been polluted by toxic prescription drugs, not to mention narcotic injections and, possibly, radiation from various brain scans. The damage these methods of pain management do to the proper functioning of the brain and nervous system, the liver and kidneys, and the cardiovascular and respiratory systems is unforgivable—not to mention that they are responsible for "rebound" headaches and buildup of drug tolerances, creating worse conditions than the original headaches you were suffering.

Headache sufferers have been gaining some control over their pain by engaging in mind/body practices such as meditation, self-hypnosis,

biofeedback, yoga, and qigong. While these methods offer a tremendous reduction in the stress-related and psychosomatic headache triggers, these encompass only a portion of headache causes, and they are
not in themselves answers to eliminating the vast spectrum of (non-
biological) headaches. Thus, no matter how many triptans you inject,
natural herbals you swallow, or needles you have stuck into your body
to control headache symptoms—like pain, nausea, and cold sweats—
the headache will surely return, leaving you to fight it another day.

The End of Suffering Is Near

I returned to the battlefield each day for twenty-seven very long years. I
lost many of the battles along the way, but without a doubt I have won
the war! In fact, I've personally gone through a plethora of "alternative" treatments for both chronic headaches and musculoskeletal pain,
including chiropractic and osteopathic manipulation, massage, Rolfing,
physical therapy, acupuncture, acupressure, qigong, Reiki, yoga, meditation, faith healing . . . you name it. I've ingested cauldrons of nasty-tasting
herbal concoctions. I've had oils rubbed onto my body, needles stuck
into my skin, energy zapped into my system, and spirits invoked over
me by shamans in trance.

As a result of these experiences and twelve years of research and
experimentation, I have come to see the headache problem as being
multi-faceted, largely self-induced, and therefore incurable by any single
healing methodology or medical model. After all, headaches are not
caused by a single factor, but by a variety of external and internal triggers;
why, then, do we expect a single treatment type to cure them? It follows,
then, that the only approach to a headache cure without adverse side effects is a comprehensive one, wherein several mind/body modalities are

integrated and led by a modification in lifestyle to effect a single end: the returning of the body to its natural, balanced state of homeostasis.

Returning the body to homeostasis can be difficult and challenging, as it may not have been in that state since birth. You see, from that point on you have been polluting it with natural and chemical toxins in the foods you eat, the beverages you drink, and the air you breathe and aggravating it with the stress you harbor and the sleep you miss. Thus, in order to reestablish homeostasis, the many toxins and stressors that tax your body must be removed or, in the case of psychosomatic triggers, dealt with in new ways. This includes being careful of the many food triggers (e.g., dairy products, red wine); correcting musculoskeletal triggers (e.g., vertebral misalignment, muscle spasms); regulating biological functions (e.g., sleeping and breathing patterns); reducing the effects of stress and anxiety; keeping the body in a perpetual state of proper hydration; and engaging in regular exercise. As you can see, for most people this approach entails a major lifestyle change. But this is truly the only way to cure headaches.

Toward a Self-Cure

The approach presented in this book is a simple one. Once you understand that your headaches are necessarily correlated with your lifestyle choices, and if you are committed to making a lasting change, then you can remove headaches from your life. Permanently!

In fact, a study conducted from 1994 to 1996 by Zuzana Bic, Dr. P.H., at Loma Linda University School of Public Health, conclusively proved that a systematic approach to migraine headache treatment using a lifestyle modification approach was effective, as long as such an approach encompassed changes in diet, exercise, and stress management.[11] She writes: "I tried the lifestyle modification approach on a group of patients diagnosed with chronic migraines. The outcome was a dramatic decrease in the frequency, intensity, and duration of headaches in over 90 percent of my patients. . . . And in many cases, patients' headaches disappeared completely."[12]

Robert Milne, M.D., and Blake More profess much of the same in their exhaustive work, *Definitive Guide to Headaches*, wherein they state: "In the majority of cases, if you pay attention and do your homework, you can identify what is causing [the headaches], eliminate the trigger from your diet, detoxify and repair your system, and, finally, live migraine free."[13]

An encompassing lifestyle change needn't be daunting or overwhelming. Things can be done in steps, one at a time. A first step is realizing that you don't have to be victim to the majority of headache attacks, especially chronic headaches. As stated earlier, most chronic headaches are caused by the foods we eat, the sleep we miss, the stresses we harbor, the tensions we embrace, the lack of water and oxygen cycled through our bodies, and by a general lack of physical exercise. In other words, they are self-induced, brought on by our own actions and indulgences.

The next step is to stop depending on or expecting your physician to "heal" you. He (or she) will not. After your physician has run the standard battery of headache tests (which is usually in the first few visits) and determined that no underlying biological cause is at the root of your pain, then nothing he can do for you will keep the headaches from coming back. Nothing! Painkillers, acupuncture, herbs, massage, whatever the treatment modality, it will only decrease the instance and symptoms of the headaches but not remove them. As long as you continue to allow headache triggers into your daily life, they will continue to do as they do: trigger headaches.

The Eight-Part Paradigm

The self-cure headache program presented here is comprehensive in its approach of integrating both Eastern and Western methods of preventing the headache triggers from taking hold through an eight-part mind/body paradigm whose sole aim is restoring the body to its natural balanced state of homeostasis. The eight parts are:

1. Drinking copious amounts of water to keep the body perpetually hydrated

2. Engaging in various methods of deep breathing to expel carbon monoxide while ensuring a continuous flow of fresh oxygen into the body

3. Detoxifying the liver, kidneys, and colon to rid the body of hazardous chemical residues and toxic buildup

4. Understanding which foods and food combinations cause headaches and how to eat around them

5. Engaging in easy walking, standing, and stretching exercises to release endorphins and work through muscle spasms while keeping the body firm and supple

6. Engaging in techniques for establishing deep and constant sleep patterns

7. Reducing the effects of stress and psychosomatic triggers on the body through various forms of meditation to quiet the mind and relax the body's nervous system

8. Having at your disposal a set of noninvasive emergency self-care remedies and methods to stop sudden headache onset in its tracks

In short, this program offers the knowledge that headaches can be prevented and, if they do occur, better managed without adverse side effects to mind or body.

The overriding premise of the integrated mind/body approach, then, is that no physician, no healer, no prayer, no mind/body methodology, and no drug by itself can prevent headaches from occurring. It is only you, the individual whose health and quality of life are at stake, who can eliminate these physically draining, emotionally stifling, and soul-destroying *forces majeure* from your life.

It is essential to understand that the information presented herein will help prevent the onset and treat the effects of migraine and cluster headaches, stress and tension headaches, allergy and sensitivity headaches, diet-induced headaches, oxygen and sleep deprivation headaches, exertion headaches, and headaches resulting from pinched nerves and other structural imbalances in the body—in other words, headaches that are *not* the result of serious head-trauma injuries or biological pathologies, such as tumors. Thankfully, as reported in the osteopathic journal *The D.O.*, "only 8 percent to 12 percent of headaches have serious underlying etiologies."[14] However, before beginning this or any other self-care program it is absolutely vital that your physician first rules out the possibility of a serious biological cause for your headache.

It is not easy to combat and triumph over the variety of headaches that attack you on a daily basis. On the contrary, it takes great courage and self-discipline to reframe your views on the subject and to maintain a healthy lifestyle for the rest of your life. But you can do it. When you have doubts, repeat these phrases:

> I am the cause of my headaches.
> I am the answer to curing my headaches.

I will not defeat myself.
I do not accept headaches in my life.
A pain-free life is my birthright!

The rest of your life starts now. Wouldn't it be great to live it pain-free and happy?

Chapter Two

UNDERSTANDING HEADACHES

If you're reading this book, you probably suffer headaches several times per month—if not weekly or daily. Chances are, so do most of the people you know. Headaches are one of the most common disorders known to man, and the human race has been suffering them since the beginning of time. Everything has been done to try to cure them, from drilling of the skull and bloodletting to prescription drug therapy and surgery. Yet headaches are still a fact of life in every country the world over.

The basic difficulty that headache sufferers face is the complexity of their problem. Not all headaches are the same, not everyone experiences headaches and their symptoms the same way, and the same stimulus (cause) does not always trigger the same type of headache. What's more, headaches encompass physical, physiological, and emotional dimensions. In short, they are multifaceted phenomena that need a comprehensive approach to achieve their banishment.

So what are headaches, what do they feel like, and what causes them? Well, according to the World Health Organizations (WHO), there are two headache types and thirteen headache classifications (along with collateral subtypes). If you have been seeing a doctor for treatment or have been doing some research, then you've probably come across a number of terms, such as migraine headache, cluster headache, tension-type headache, allergy headache, sinus headache, and so on. While such classifications are a good way to start, the problem is that they never tell the whole story.

As an example, depending on circumstances you may be experiencing two or more different types of headaches at one time. This happens because one stimulus can trigger more than one headache type, and one headache type can trigger another, and so on. That is why the medication you took for your headache yesterday worked, while today it doesn't seem to be helping at all. Adding to the confusion, many headaches present the same symptoms, such as shaking, fever, throbbing or pulsating pain, tight muscles, hypersensitive nerves, listlessness, vomiting, and so on. Thus, trying to identify and distinguish them based on symptoms can be frustrating, nearly impossible in some cases, and, in a word, useless. As a headache sufferer, it is only important to know why you are getting headaches and how to stop them from happening again.

This chapter is concerned with understanding headaches rather than treating them, so I will begin by outlining a few things that may give you deeper insight into your pain. First, we'll look at major headache types and their symptoms, as they are generally viewed by practitioners of Western medicine. Then we'll take up the concept of energy pathways and their correlation with the organs and quadrants of the head, as viewed by practitioners of Traditional Chinese Medicine. Finally, I will provide an outline and description of the most common (and infamous) headache causes or triggers—which, as a headache sufferer, you should be mindful to avoid at all times.

Headache Types and Categories: A Western Perspective

In 1988, the International Headache Classification was developed and published by the International Headache Society. This system has been adopted by the World Health Organizations and is now the main reference for diagnosis and treatment of headache among Western-trained physicians. While the list is specific as needed for Western methods of diagnosis and treatment, for our *self-directed integrated mind/body approach toward a self-cure*, the following grouping of two types and eight categories is sufficient.

In essence, all headaches can be identified as being either *primary* or *secondary*. Primary headaches are those in which the headache pain itself is the problem, and these include all headaches aside from those with an organic origin. Secondary headaches are the direct result of an underlying medical problem, such as a virus, brain tumor, meningitis, or recent head trauma. In other words, the headache is a symptom of a larger, perhaps life-threatening problem.

The shortcoming of this two-type model of headache is that it assumes *all* headaches can be regarded as symptoms that something is not right in the body. While there may be no organic disease causing the headache, certainly there is something triggering it, such as excessive toxins in the body, dehydration, chronic stress, or lack of sleep, for example. All headaches, then, can be considered secondary since something cannot be created from nothing. What's more, all (nonorganic) headaches are self-induced to a large extent, and therefore curable with the proper lifestyle modification.

Let us now take a look at some of the headache classifications so we can get a more general idea of what triggers specific types of headaches and what type of symptoms they cause. Since many of the headache categories in the classification list have overlapping triggers and symptoms, I am grouping them here in somewhat broader terms.

ORGANIC HEADACHES

Headaches that are the result of an underlying biological problem are classified as *organic.* While these headaches are indeed rare, they are potentially the most lethal and must, under all circumstances, be ruled out before attempting to treat your head pain in any fashion. Headaches that are classified as organic include those caused by meningitis, encephalitis, multiple sclerosis, diseased blood vessels, concussions, stroke, epilepsy, brain tumor, bleeding aneurysm, and other serious disorders.

(As stated earlier, the integrated mind/body approach outlined in this book will not prevent or reduce symptoms associated with organic headaches.)

CLUSTER HEADACHES

While they are less life-threatening than organic headaches, and less common than migraines, cluster headaches are without doubt the most painful and difficult to deal with, as they occur in "clusters" or in-tervals of time and days.

Affecting roughly one million Americans, 90 percent of them male, cluster headaches are vascular in nature and are distinguished by their attacks, which last for only a few hours at a time but keep recurring over the course of several days or even a month.[1] The pain is generally clustered around or behind one eye or temple and is akin to an object being jammed into the eye. Symptoms include a steady sharp pain, tearing and nasal congestion, reddening of the affected eye, and sweating. Unlike migraines, cluster headaches do not present nausea, vomiting, or sensitivity to light—although, in my experience, when accompanied with migraine, death feels like a viable option.

While the direct cause of cluster headaches is not certain, research supports the theory that it may originate in the part of the brain known as the hypothalamus, which affects levels of neurotransmitters such as serotonin. However, researchers do know that these headaches are vascular, and as such they can be triggered by alcohol, food, caffeine, extreme temperatures, and changes of season.[2]

MIGRAINE HEADACHES

Chronic migraine headaches are incapacitating, traumatic events in the lives of twenty-six million headache sufferers in the United States. Migraine headaches are of the vascular type, as they are believed to be associated with the constriction and expansion of blood vessels in the head and are categorized as either *classic* or *common*. Classic migraine is usually associated with the presence of a view-obstructing aura some 30 minutes or so prior to an attack. Common migraines are not accompanied or preceded by an aura, but they are no less painful.

Migraine sufferers usually describe their pain as throbbing or pounding on one side of the head in tandem with their pulse, which changes to a steady sharp or blinding pain, with numbness in the affected area and featuring general somatic weakness. Attacks usually last as briefly as several hours or as long as three or more days and are generally accompanied by trembling, sweating, and vomiting. During attacks, sufferers tend to be hypersensitive to light, sounds, and smells and often desire to be left alone in quiet rooms with the blankets pulled over their heads and ice packs on their temples.

Migraines can be triggered by a number of things, the most common of which are low levels of serotonin in the blood, too little or too much sleep, hunger or overeating, changes in blood sugar and blood fat levels, food or chemical allergies, toxic buildup in the intestine, and constipation.

MUSCLE-CONTRACTION HEADACHES

Muscle-contraction headaches (also known as tension-type headaches) are both the most common and least debilitating of all headaches and are said to account for approximately 90 percent of all headaches.[3] They are so-named because of the excessive muscle tension in the head, neck, and shoulders associated with them that irritate head and facial nerves and thus cause pain.

Muscle-contraction headaches are classified as being either chronic (repeated) or episodic (sporadic), and they generally last anywhere from a few minutes to a few hours or even several days. They are characterized by a stiff neck and shoulders and a dull, achy pain in the head, temples, and forehead that feels as if a band were being squeezed around the head.

While annoying, these headaches do not necessarily hamper daily life functions. For those who are prone to them, they can be triggered by a great many things, including stress and anxiety, eyestrain, poor posture, structural misalignment (including TMJ), and sleep deprivation. Tension headaches tend to subside quickly when their trigger is removed.

EXERTION HEADACHES

Exertion headaches are also quite common among those who are susceptible to getting headaches. These can either be triggered by the sudden spurt of energy or prolonged use of muscles. Exertion headaches tend to present throbbing or pounding pain and are often short in duration. They generally occur when one sits up quickly after laying prone for some time, after a strenuous exertion when lifting or pushing a heavy object, straining while going to the bathroom, or during sexual intercourse. In other words, abdominal contraction combined with the holding of the breath and physical exertion can cause exertion headaches.

According to the research of Robert Milne, M.D., and Blake More, exertion headaches are a type of vascular headache. Current theories suggest that they cause pain because swelling in the arteries and veins forces the blood vessels in the head and scalp to swell.[4]

ALLERGY/SENSITIVITY HEADACHES

Once upon a time, doctors associated migraines with allergies and also misdiagnosed them as sinus headaches, since they share common symptoms. However, despite heavy product marketing to the contrary, sinus headaches are very rare. In fact, what distinguishes them is prolonged facial pain, thick mucus, and fever. While the above two suppositions have since been disproved, many headaches have an underlying food, chemical, or environmental allergy or sensitivity at their root.

For those who are prone to getting them, triggers for allergy/ sensitivity headaches can include stress, food, light, cigarette smoke, pollen, alcohol, pesticides—almost anything. Pain associated with allergy headaches is generally dull and diffused over the entire head, with no easily identifiable locus. Such headaches are known to come on several hours after contact with the problematic substance, and are easy to offset by simply removing the thing that caused the allergic reaction.[5]

REBOUND/RECUPERATIVE HEADACHES

Rebound headaches are so named because they occur as the body "rebounds" from overconsumption or withdrawal from too many analgesics or prescription medications, coffee or caffeine-laden soft drinks, or alcohol. They are also caused by elevated adrenaline levels, sleep disorders, and so on.

Like migraine and cluster headaches, rebound headaches are vascular in nature and characterized by steady pounding or throbbing on both sides of the head caused by constricting and dilating blood vessels. This type of vascular headache is in theory the easiest to prevent, but since it is directly triggered by poor lifestyle choices, it may be the most difficult to eliminate. In essence, rebound headaches are a recuperative measure whereby the body is telling you by way of head pain that something is wrong and forcing rest and change in behavior. Rebound headaches occur commonly as a result of toxic buildup of medication, alcohol, or caffeine in the system, as well as from prolonged periods of physically draining activity, such as cramming for finals or that wild weekend party that left you with a hangover.

Here's what Oliver Sacks, M.D., has to say about them: "There is usually a rather sharp collapse from the preceding or provocative period of overactivity and tension. . . . Recuperative attacks have the closest biological analogy to sleep, and are clearly preservative reflexes."[6]

Now we know that not all headaches are alike, and we know how each type of headache is experienced and affects us in a different way. Let's take a moment to look at a system of traditional healing that gives specific meaning to where the headache originates.

Headache Locations and Patterns:
An Eastern Perspective

Traditional Chinese Medicine (TCM) views the human body as an integrated and organic whole that cannot be separated from nature. In short, every part of a human being—be it organ, cell, muscle, or thought—is inseparable from and influenced by every other part, and a problem with one part in turn affects the function of every other part. Therefore, headaches aren't seen as a set of symptoms reduced to a specific disease as they are in Western thinking, but rather they're viewed as merely a part (or symptom) of an overall pattern of imbalance in the body. Once the pattern of disharmony is balanced, its resultant symptoms (e.g., headache, blurred vision, anxiety) will disappear. In essence, TCM believes that there are only three causes of illness: excess, stagnation, or deficiency of vital energy and fluids in the body.

In my research toward understanding my own headaches and eventually curing myself of them, I found that the fundamentals of TCM acquainted me with these monsters in a new and enlightening way. As you will come to see by the end of this chapter, it is the TCM model of disease cause and treatment that was in large part responsible for the formation of the *integrated mind/body approach to headache prevention* presented in this book.

FUNDAMENTAL THEORIES OF TCM

Traditional Chinese Medicine is both an art and a science. It is founded on a set of fundamental theories which East Asian physicians apply as they try to understand the pattern of disharmony that is the underlying cause of any illness or disease. These theories include *yin* and *yang*, the five elements; the *zang-fu* organ system, the four substances, and the energy meridian channels. Each is described in brief below.

Yin and yang—The Taoist theory of *yin* and *yang* holds that the world is composed of two opposing yet complementary forces: positive and negative. Originally, these forces were conceived of metaphorically as water and fire. All things that hold the properties of water (feminine, cold, still, nurturing, downward) are considered *yin*, while those things that possess the attributes of fire (masculine, hot, moving, destructive, upward) are considered *yang*. Everything in the macrocosmic world, then, can be seen as either *yin* or *yang*. One cannot exist without the other; thus the two are interdependent. As examples, there can be no sense of what is hot without first knowing what is cold; there can be no feeling of failure without first knowing success; there can be no up without a down.

In TCM, the structure and inner functions of the human body is seen as a *microcosm* of the world, and as such, all aspects are divided into *yin* and *yang*. This also means that every aspect of the body relates to and is affected by every other aspect. In these terms, the upper and exterior parts of the body are considered *yang*, while the lower and interior parts are considered *yin*. Even within each division, there is further subdivision. As such, the heart, lungs, spleen, liver, and kidneys belong to *yin*, while the gallbladder, stomach, small and large intestines, and urinary bladder are ascribed to *yang*. It is believed that the separation of *yin* and *yang* can only lead to death.

The five elements—The theory of the five elements holds that the world is metaphorically composed of five basic elements: wood, fire, earth, metal, and water. As with *yin* and *yang*, every aspect and function of the human body is ascribed to one of these basic elements, and this is used to explain the etiology and pathogenesis of illness. This system also informs the physician how to treat and prevent disease from taking hold in the body. These elements, furthermore, are believed to mutually promote and restrict one another. For example: wood produces (generates) fire, while fire produces earth (in the form of ashes). Conversely, water restricts (extinguishes) fire, while earth restricts (absorbs) water. Thus we have interdependent promotion and restriction among the five elements, and this is important to understand the physiology of the body and the pathology of an illness, such as headaches.

The *zang-fu* organ system—In TCM, the organs of the body are known as *zang* (organ) and *fu* (bowel), and they are each believed to hold the characteristics of *yin* or *yang* and one of the five elements, based on the specific organ's form and function. As examples, the spleen is thought to possess the attributes of *yin* (feminine) and earth (generating) since it produces blood and nourishes the body; the bladder, conversely, is thought of as *yang* (masculine) and water (flowing) since it is active in its removal of liquid waste from the body. Moreover, every organ is thought to control a specific emotion, and each *zang* organ is paired with a specific *fu* organ. Therefore, we find the kidneys and urinary bladder as a *yin/yang* pair, wherein an impairment of one affects the function of the other. Have you ever been so scared that you wet your pants? This happens because fear and fright harm the kidney, causing its qi (vital or intrinsic energy) to flow downward, thus causing reflexive urination and/or loss of bowel control.

The four substances—TCM further holds that the body is controlled and we are kept alive by four basic substances known as essence, *qi*, blood, and body fluids. The absence of any one of these would prevent normal body functions from being carried out, and so an excess, stagnation, or deficiency of any of them can lead to pain, illness, or disease.

Essence *(jing)* is described as the material basis responsible for the physiological functions of the human body. *Qi* is believed to be the very particles that compose the universe and everything in it. It is the energy and force produced by these particles that is responsible for the overall function of the human body. While there are several forms of *qi*, they all relate to energetic functions in and of the body, and this *qi* is acquired mostly from the air we breathe and the food and beverages we drink. Therefore, poor diet and poor breathing patterns lead to disharmony and dysfunction of the body. Have you ever eaten a nutritionally deprived lunch of fried food and sugary soda, only to find yourself quickly out of energy with difficulty breathing and soon lying down with a pounding headache? This happens because poor diet equals poor *qi*, and poor *qi* equals poor health and the onset of any number of types of headaches.

Energy meridian channels—While all of these things thus far seem, well, *foreign* to many of us, there is actually a thread that connects and unifies them, and this is the system of energy channels commonly known in the West as meridians. TCM holds that the body is composed of a network of twelve regular and eight collateral channels, or energy pathways, through which *qi* and blood circulate. Each regular channel is named after the specific organ it relates to, and each channel exists bilaterally in the body. These channels are the mechanism that moves intrinsic energy and blood throughout the body, connecting the *zang* (*yin*) organs with the *fu* (*yang*) organs, with the musculoskeletal system, with the respiratory system, with the skin and hair and orifices of the body— thus ensuring that we remain an organic (healthy) whole.

ETIOLOGY OF ILLNESS AND DISEASE

The epigraph that opens this book is so important and profound in terms of understanding headache cause and cure that I present it again here: *Tong ze be tong; Bu tong ze tong*—If there is free flow, there is no

pain; If there is pain, there is no free flow. In terms of TCM, pain, illness, and disease only surface when there is either an excess, stagnation,
or deficiency in the production, flow, and removal of the four basic substances of existence: essence, *qi*, blood, and body fluids.

What causes these substances to come to excess, stagnation, or deficiency? The Chinese believe that the harmonious balance (homeostasis) of *yin/yang*, five elements, *zang-fu* organs, four essential substances,
and the meridian complex is disrupted by either external or internal
pathogenic factors. The external factors are known as the six pernicious
influences, and they include: wind, cold, summer heat, damp, dryness,
and fire. When your immune system is weak, these climatic factors are
able to invade the meridians and cause illness and disease—including
headache.

The primary internal factor leading to illness is excess of one or
more of the seven emotions: joy, anger, melancholy, anxiety, grief, fear,
and fright. Do you recall a time when you were so angry that it felt as if
your blood was boiling, and your eyes turned red and a devastating
headache was soon upon you? This happens because anger causes heat
in the liver, which causes liver *qi* and blood to rise upward (as opposed
to the liver energy's normal downward movement), causing the face
and eyes to turn red and the top of the head to ache.

The Chinese also hold that lifestyle choices can directly lead to disease, and these include an excess or deficient diet, physical and sexual
activity, rest and sleep, and work and play. In other words, too much of
one and too little of another leads to disharmony of *yin* and *yang*—and
when *yin* and *yang* separate, illness results.

When there is a blockage (stagnation) in a meridian, symptoms are
sure to develop, as the energy cannot pass between organs and parts of
the body. Have you ever felt pain in your shoulder and later in the day
experienced a headache in the back of your head? How about a

stomach cramp or constipation where you later experienced what you thought was an unrelated frontal headache? This happens because after birth we derive the majority of our *qi* from what the ancient Chinese physicians called "water and grain." Therefore, lack of food, too much food, or heavy and fatty foods can lead to malfunction of the stomach, which causes *qi* and blood moving in the stomach meridian to a position of excess, stagnation, or deficiency—thus causing pain in the head.

DIAGNOSIS AND TREATMENT PRINCIPLES

Unlike his biomedical counterpart, the physician of Traditional Chinese Medicine does not toss a host of symptoms into a funnel and hope that from the bottom emerges a specific disease to name and treat. In contrast, the doctor of Oriental medicine gathers information directly and indirectly from the patient and, in his attempt to see the body as an integrated organic whole, comes to see a pattern of disharmony.

This pattern of disharmony is comprised of irregularities in the patient discovered through what is termed the four examinations: inspection (observation of vitality, color, appearance, five sense organs, tongue), auscultation and olfaction (listening and smelling), inquiring (asking about chills and fever, perspiration, appetite, thirst, taste, bowel function, pain, sleep, menses, etc.), and palpation (feeling several pulses along the radial artery and palpating different parts of the body).

From the four examinations, the doctor of Chinese medicine will consider the eight principle patterns (*yin/yang*, hot/cold, interior/exterior, and deficiency/excess) and determine what the pattern of disharmony is in the patient and which organs/meridians are affected. In terms of headaches, four of the six main meridian channels (or eight of the twelve, if you count them bilaterally) travel directly to specific areas of the head. Therefore, in terms of Traditional Chinese Medicine, the following is held to be true:

✦ Headaches that are felt to originate on the vertex or top of the head are directly related to the functions of the liver and pericardium.

✦ Headaches that are experienced on the forehead are directly related to the functions of the stomach and large intestines.

✦ Headaches that grip the occipital or back of the head are directly related to the functions of the small intestines and urinary bladder.

✦ Headaches that are felt across the temples or around the head like a band are directly related to the functions of the heart and kidneys.

I know that all of this can sound confusing, so I offer the following example with the hope that it will better illustrate how the components of TCM fit together.

Amanda is a copywriter with a hectic daily schedule. Her workload is often daunting and her deadlines loom ominously, so she takes her work home and is only able to sleep a few hours each night. This leaves Amanda exhausted, and after several weeks of this, her productivity becomes substandard, which forces her to rewrite several projects. This, of course, leads her to miss a few deadlines. Management is unhappy, and stress becomes prevalent. Amanda's boss summons her to the office for a lecture, which she resents, and in an attempt at self-preservation, she says nothing in her defense—only harboring ill feelings, anger, and a little resentment. Happy hour is her way out, her release from stress, and the only way she can unwind each day. The weekend comes and Amanda notices, as she reaches for the Excedrin bottle, that it is nearly empty—yet she just purchased it late last week. When her body has a chance to rest, she realizes that her head has been pounding for a week without let-up, and that she has been too busy to fully acknowledge either the headache or her new dependence on analgesics.

According to TCM, stress, anger, and alcohol all cause too much qi to gather in the body, thus creating excess heat that adversely affects the functions of the liver. Liver heat is *yang,* and too much *yang* means there is too little *yin,* causing a kidney (water element) *yin* deficiency which cannot properly generate or nourish the liver (wood element). Since heat rises, this excess qi ascends upward, causing a headache at the vertex or top of the head, where the liver meridians travel. The eyes may be painful and bloodshot because they are, according to Traditional Chinese Medicine, the outlet of the liver.

More specifically, in terms of the five element theory, wood (the liver) derives nourishment from water (the kidneys). If the kidneys become deficient in *yin* as a result of excess *yang,* the liver is affected with a heat *(yang)* excess. And since wood (the liver) restricts earth (the stomach), too much heat in the liver may cause excess heat in the stomach as well, thus leading to another headache on the front of the head, where the stomach meridians travel. However, since metal (the lungs) control or restrict wood (the liver), a simple way of aborting the rise in liver *yang* is to sit for a time in a state of slow and controlled deep breathing. This induces the relaxation response by releasing held tensions and feelings, thus allowing *yin* to balance *yang.* (For more information on TCM and headaches, I highly recommend the book *Migraines and Traditional Chinese Medicine* by Bob Flaws.[7]

With all these things in mind, the TCM physician will, depending on the headache location, treat the patient with a single modality or a combination of acupuncture, moxibustion (the warming of acupoints with moxa cones or moxa wool), herbal formulas, qigong (energy therapy), or tuina (bodywork therapy). He or she may also recommend lifestyle changes in terms of sleep, work habits, diet, and so on.

However, it is still up to the patient—the headache sufferer—to prevent the archnemesis from returning time and again. Although the doctor or healer can remove symptoms for a short period of time, it is only the headache sufferer himself or herself who can prevent them from taking hold once more by making informed lifestyle choices and following *the integrated mind/body approach.*

Headache Causes and Triggers

Now you have basic knowledge that there are many different types and categories of headaches, as defined in terms of the Western medical model. You also know, as seen in the East Asian medical model, that headaches are caused only by excess, stagnation, or deficiency in the body, and that the part of the head affected directly relates to specific organ functions or at least to the meridian channels associated with those organs. You also know that you don't necessarily get the same type of headache every time, and oftentimes they attack in combination, which is why ibuprofin diminishes the pain sometimes and not at others.

Let us now look at some of the things known to trigger headaches, so that we can be careful to avoid their excess and thus prevent the onset of headaches in the future. The chapters that follow will present an in-depth look at the most important triggers and how to remove or prevent them—permanently. Here, however, is an overview to better illustrate the headache spectrum.

OXYGEN DEPRIVATION AND CHRONIC DEHYDRATION

The two most important elements to human existence are oxygen and water. Without them, we would cease to exist. While both are in great abundance, the majority of people neither breathe properly nor consume adequate amounts of water to satisfy basic bodily needs and functions. Multitudes of studies have confirmed that low levels of both water and oxygen in the body can trigger migraine and cluster headaches.

IMPROPER BIOCHEMICAL LEVELS

For the body to function at homeostasis, all its chemicals must be at proper levels. However, when levels of certain chemicals drop or rise, they can trigger various types of headaches. Low levels of the neurotransmitter serotonin, high levels of fats in the blood, low blood sugar, high levels of histamine, and low levels of magnesium, vitamins A and C, and the B vitamins are all known headache triggers. Regulating these chemicals in the body and maintaining those levels is a key factor in preventing certain types of headaches.

FOOD AND CHEMICAL SENSITIVITIES

For people who are prone to them, headaches resulting from food, chemical, and environmental sensitivities or allergies can become a chronic problem. The chemicals found in the tap water we drink and the pesticide residues and hormones in the foods we eat can trigger headaches. Specific types of foods, such as aged cheese, red wine, tomato sauce, pickled foods, dairy products, cocoa, alcohol, and caffeine, are known culprits. Learning how to avoid the sensitivities and changing your eating habits will do much to eliminate those triggers.

INADEQUATE EXERCISE AND REST

Endorphins are the body's natural painkillers, and they are released during prolonged physical activity. One of the major causes of headaches is inactivity. Aside from lowering oxygen intake and endorphin levels in the body, a host of other diseases result from lack of exercise. A sedentary lifestyle also assists in the creation of imbalances in the musculoskeletal system, which can trigger certain types of headaches. And for those who do exercise, or who don't but who are workaholics, inadequate rest and sleep can also cause headaches by not allowing the body to rejuvenate itself.

MUSCULOSKELETAL IMBALANCES

Imbalances in both the muscular and skeletal systems can lead to headaches in a number of ways. Misaligned vertebrae can irritate nerves, sending pain signals to the head. Nerve sensitivity and muscle spasms in the back, shoulders, and neck can cause muscle-contraction or tension-type headaches. Improper posture while seated or standing, ergonomically incorrect positions when typing or playing the piano, for example, also lead to musculoskeletal imbalances and then to headaches. When combined, moderate exercise, postural correction, and proper stretching can correct such imbalances to the musculoskeletal system and thus prevent such triggers from causing headaches.

THE MIND IN THE BODY

The mind has a tremendous, if nonspecific, influence on the body. In medical terms, illnesses and diseases originating from the mind/body connection are known as psychosomatic. Stress, anxiety, depression, poor posture, lack of sleep, and poor eating habits are all psychosomatic indications that can trigger a number of headaches in a number of ways. Our mind is perhaps our greatest enemy when it comes to headaches. Coming to understand the mind/body connection in the cause and prevention of headaches will be a great advantage in ridding you of these monsters once and for all.

Chapter Three

OXYGEN AND HEADACHE

Oxygen is the single most important element to humans. Without air to breathe we would cease to exist. Indeed, life begins with the first breath and ends with the last. Yet, while our planet provides us with ample quantities of oxygen, few of us take full advantage of it. That is, we breathe shallowly, filling only a small percentage of our lung capacity—and this is making us unhealthy.

The Chinese have a saying, and I paraphrase: When we're born, we instinctively breathe deeply with our abdomen; as adults, we tend to breathe from our chests; as we near death, we breathe only from our throats. In other words, the less full and more superficial our breathing, the closer to death we become. And while we of course do not breathe from our stomachs, the act of expanding and contracting the abdomen while breathing facilitates a full and complete breathing cycle by drawing fresh air to the bottom of the lungs and expelling stale air from the same region.

How Oxygen Deprivation Causes Headaches

Though we don't consciously think of it, the way we breathe has a direct effect on our state of health and well-being, with the power to either make us ill or to heal us. Have you ever been so scared that you forgot to breathe, like when a car suddenly pulled out in front of you? How about the last time you were feeling stressed out? If you were too busy or preoccupied to do something about it, your breath became short and labored, and this perhaps led to your getting a dull, pounding headache. If you took a moment to draw in a few deep breaths, you could have become instantly more relaxed and your breathing cycle would have become steady, thus averting the headache.

Proper breathing allows many vital life functions to occur, including filling the body with ample levels of oxygen to feed the blood and brain, to burn food and release energy, and to expel toxic carbon monoxide with each exhalation. Yawning is a sure sign that our bodies are lacking in oxygen, as the process brings in a deep breath of air in one instant. Not only is yawning a sure sign that our bodies are in need of more oxygen, it may also be a sign that an oxygen-deprivation headache may be on its way. Shallow breathing occurs when you are tired, under stress, or have been sitting still for a long time.

Without an ample supply of oxygen in our lungs, our cells, tissues, and organs will be unable to function properly. When this happens, toxins and histamines are allowed to build up in our bloodstreams, and vascular headaches (such as migraine and cluster) are the result. This happens because low oxygen levels force a widening of the blood vessels in an effort to allow more blood to flow through them, thus causing headaches. In order to prevent this, more oxygen must be supplied to the brain. The best way to do this is by deep breathing and by increasing your levels of physical activity.[1]

People who either snore when they sleep, sleep with their heads face-down on their pillows, or sleep in areas with poor ventilation are susceptible to getting cluster headaches that result from low levels of oxygen in their blood and brains. At the advice and prescription of their doctors, some sufferers of oxygen-deprivation headaches keep a tank of pure oxygen by their beds and inhale the air through a mask to abort a cluster headache in progress. Inhaling pure oxygen has been clinically proven to decrease cluster headaches by as much as 80 percent.[2]

The shortcoming of these methods, again, is that we are dealing with treating headache symptoms after they have occurred, rather than preventing them in the first place. As should be your mantra by now, such after-the-fact pain-relief methods will never prevent the headaches and their symptoms from arising. In short, oxygen-deprivation headaches are the result of our own lack of proper breathing.

Andrew Weil, M.D., is among the few Western-trained physicians who professes the many healing powers of proper breathing as part of a comprehensive wellness program. I highly recommend his work, as well as that of Jon Kabat-Zinn, Ph.D., Herbert Benson, M.D., and Daniel Goleman, Ph.D., whose respective research on breathing and meditative states has revolutionized mind/body medicine in the United States.

The program advocated in this book is one of self-regulation. A sufficient intake of oxygen requires only that we breathe correctly, and that we use deep-breathing techniques when stress and tensions begin to arise in our bodies, leading to slower blood flow and oxygen-deprivation headaches. Proper, deep breathing increases levels of oxygen in the lungs, improving respiratory functions and oxygen levels in the blood, thus improving delivery of oxygen to the cells.

Full breathing brings more oxygen into the head and nourishes the central nervous system. As a result, the blood vessels of the skin constrict, blood pressure drops slightly, and peripheral blood flow slows. This establishes a harmonious pattern for other bodily rhythms and also regulates moods and emotions—all events that help prevent headaches.[3]

Self-Regulating Breathing Exercises

Proper breathing depends on filling the lungs to their full capacity. Deep-breathing practices have been embraced by Eastern mystics and healers for thousands of years, as evidenced in breath-work's major standing in yoga and qigong practices. In fact, a study on deep breathing in India revealed that after 15 minutes of practice, the average volume of air taken into the lungs on inhalation rose from 482 ml before practice to 740 ml afterward, while the average number of breaths per minute dropped from fifteen down to five. This represents a huge improvement in respiratory efficiency.[4]

To help prevent headache triggers and reduce their symptoms of pain, nausea, and shortness of breath, I recommend the following program of four exercises. These are simple yet highly effective exercises originating from yoga and qigong.

ABDOMINAL BREATHING

This exercise will help you get the feel for proper breathing.

1. Lie down on your back, with knees bent and feet flat on the floor a foot's distance from your buttocks.

2. With your lower back resting on the floor, inhale deeply, taking in a full breath of air.

3. If you allow your abdomen to rise (expand) as you inhale, you will be able to fill your lungs to capacity. If you allow your abdomen to sink (contract) on exhale, you will be able to fully expel all of the air (fresh and stale) from the lowermost quadrants of your lungs.

4. Repeat this no less than a dozen times during each cycle.

5. Try to be mindful of the experience as a whole while engaging in it.

NOSTRIL BREATHING WITH SOUND

A fundamental method for beginning proper breathing is to open and fully utilize both nostrils. The following exercise is known as *ujjayi* breathing, or breathing with sound. It helps overcome tension and vitalizes the body in general and the nervous system in particular. It can also relieve depression and may induce deeper states of consciousness. The exercise described here is that taught at the SKY Yoga Foundation and the Yoga Research Society as led by Vijayendra Pratap, Ph.D., D.Y.P.[5]

1. Sit in a comfortable position.

2. Raise the chest first while inhaling, then expand the rib cage, and then the abdomen. Keep the abdomen slightly contracted.

3. Follow the reverse order in exhalation: contract the abdomen, rib cage, and finally the chest, but without too much movement of the chest.

4. Keeping with the tradition, inhale through both nostrils, retain the breath, and then exhale through the left nostril.

5. Take the breath in with a partial closure of the glottis, as a person does in snoring, but in a smooth, rhythmic, controlled way. The inhalation should last 8 counts.

6. Retain or hold the breath for a count of 32. While doing this, place your thumb at the right nostril, keeping the ring finger and little finger at the bridge of the nose, preferably with the ring finger touching the point between the eyebrows.

7. Exhale with sound for a count of 16. You can learn to produce the proper sound by exhaling through your mouth with a "ha" sound, then do the same with your mouth closed.

8. Close your eyes and attend to the sound you produce.

9. Repeat 10 times or so, increasing gradually only if you are comfortable.

The Chinese have also fostered good health and long life by developing hundreds of breathing and energy exercises known under the rubric of qigong, which translates literally as "breath work." Qigong is actually more than just breath work, as it encompasses a dynamic interplay and connection of breath, spirit, intrinsic energy, intention, body posture, and movement sequences. While there are traditionally five categories or schools of qigong practice (Taoist, Buddhist, Confucian, medical, and martial), their goal is the same: a healthy unity of mind and body through the development and control of *qi* or intrinsic energy. Stricken of its archaic symbolism and terms, *qi* can best be described as the harnessing and directed flow of electromagnetic energy in the body through breath, visualization, and movement exercises as directed by the mind.

Qigong master FaXiang Hou and the Qigong Research Society have proven that a daily practice of 15 minutes a day of the following qigong exercises can prevent headaches caused by oxygen deprivation, poor blood flow, vascular dilation, stress, tension, and digestive problems.[6]

CHEST BREATHING

1. Stand in a comfortable position with shoulders relaxed, hands by your sides, legs a shoulder's width apart.

2. Close your eyes and make sure your neck, shoulders, arms, and legs are relaxed.

3. Inhale through your nose evenly and quietly, pulling oxygen into your lungs, expanding them to full capacity. Be sure to inflate the chest only, and not the stomach.

4. Exhale slightly longer than the inhalation, and as you do so push the stale breath out through your mouth slowly, evenly, and quietly. Be sure to contract your chest and lungs to their least capacity.

5. You may perform this exercise as often as you like throughout the day, but not for more than 5 minutes at any one time.

UPPER-STOMACH BREATHING

1. Stand in a comfortable position, with shoulders relaxed, hands by your sides, legs a shoulder's width apart.

2. Close your eyes and make sure your neck, shoulders, arms, and legs are relaxed.

3. Inhale through your nose evenly and quietly, pulling oxygen into the area between the navel and diaphragm. Be sure to expand the upper stomach only to full capacity, and not the chest or lower stomach areas.

4. Exhale slightly longer than inhalation, and as you do so push the stale air out through your mouth slowly, evenly, and quietly.

5. Many people find this area of their body difficult to isolate while breathing, but if you remain loose, relaxed, and focused you can do it and the health benefits will come.

Proper breathing exercises are more than just methods of increasing overall oxygen consumption in the lungs and flow through the blood and to the brain; they also work effectively to reduce the onset of headaches with psychosomatic triggers (i.e., those related to and caused by an imbalance in mind and body). Deep breathing has the power to alter consciousness, calm the mind, center the spirit, and relax tense muscles. While Eastern mystics have been utilizing breathing methods for thousands of years, for all our great advances in medical science it is only in the past thirty years that Western-trained physicians have been incorporating them into their treatments.

Once you experience the feeling of deep breathing, you will be able to do it at any time your body may cue you to do so—such as when tensions seize your shoulders and spine, or when your breath becomes shallow from stress and anxiety due to deadline-driven workloads, or when you feel a dull, pounding headache caused by shallow breathing.

Proper breathing is not only the key to good health, but it is also a sure way of preventing some of headache's most notorious triggers from taking hold in your body. So relax, take some deep breaths, and discover how great you will begin to feel.

Chapter Four

DEHYDRATION AND HEADACHE

It is vital that every human being drink copious amounts of water every day—especially those who suffer headaches. Since water makes up roughly 75 percent or three-fourths of the human body (and 85 percent of the brain), it only makes sense that no tissue, organ, or gland can function properly without ample supply of this natural fluid. It is the improper functioning of the digestive system, lungs, liver, and kidneys that not only contributes to and triggers headaches, but makes us ill. Indeed, we humans would surely cease to exist without the magic elixir known as water, which, next to oxygen, is the most vital substance on Earth.

Drinking ample quantities of water every day is so important that for centuries many traditional cultures have engaged its healing qualities to cure and prevent various illnesses and diseases. Traditional Chinese medicine, for example, recognized the healing powers of water more than three thousand years ago. Even Hippocrates, the father of modern Medicine, was said to have drunk and bathed in water to benefit from the healing properties of its mineral content.[1] Indeed, the mere consumption of this fluid can help restore the body to its natural state of homeostasis by clearing toxins, cleansing the colon, flushing the liver and kidneys, and emptying the bowels—all necessary functions to removing and preventing a number of headaches.

How Dehydration Causes Headaches

With the relative abundance of water available in the United States and the sheer necessity of it to our health and well-being, it is a wonder how many illnesses and ailments suffered by Americans—including headaches—are actually caused or aggravated by simple dehydration. The leading researcher of our time on illness and diseases caused by dehydration is F. Batmanghelidj, M.D., an internist trained at St. Mary's Hospital Medical School of London University and one of the last students of Sir Alexander Fleming, the discoverer of penicillin. In his book, *Your Body's Many Cries for Water*, Dr. Batmanghelidj asserts that "Chronic, unintentional dehydration is the origin of most pain and degenerative diseases in the human body."[2] These, he notes, include migraines.

It was while spending several years as a political prisoner in an Iranian prison that Dr. Batmanghelidj came to discover the healing powers of simple water, and the negative effects of dehydration. While his research has been focused on such chronic illnesses as heartburn, lupus, arthritis, and peptic ulcers, in an interview published at PhenomeNEWS.com he stated that migraines are " . . . a sign of water need by the brain and the eyes. They will totally clear up if dehydration is prevented from establishing in the body."[3]

Batmanghelidj found that as the water content of tissues falls to a certain point as a result of dehydration, the bi-layer membranes that surround cells contract, forming a barrier that prevents further water loss. This obstructs the free movement of molecules, so that metabolism and elimination are limited. Slow metabolism and elimination lead to buildup of toxins in the blood, which can manifest as a chemical-induced headache.

It is important to understand that regardless of the quantity of your daily water intake, its percentage in urine remains constant at around 95 percent. When the hypothalamus detects a lowering of water volume in the body, it signals the pituitary gland to release the antidiuretic hormone (ADH) into the bloodstream, which increases the capacity of the kidneys to reabsorb and recycle water. In essence, when the body moves into survival mode by contracting the bi-layer membranes, the kidneys keep recycling and concentrating the urine in an effort to maintain sufficient hydration. Thus, the less water put into the body, the less the body's ability to cleanse itself of poisonous toxins through elimination via urine, feces, perspiration, and the breath. And since waste products left to accumulate in your tissues create chronic pain, headaches, and many diseases, water intake is necessary to facilitate the effective elimination of the toxic buildup.

It is in part due to overtaxing the colonic tract by overeating, ingesting foods high in spices, nitrates, and other chemical content, and taking in an abundance of sugars or alcohol, that we feel exhausted, lethargic, experience seemingly unending dull headaches, catch colds easily, or become seriously ill. It is the absorption of the nutrients in the colon and intestines from the food we eat that prevents, causes, or cures what ails us. In fact, research has indicated that a thorough flushing of the mucus folds in the colonic tract where toxins and wastes generally remain will cleanse the system and keep the body healthy and the immune system strong. At the same time, quantities of water are known to revitalize the kidney and liver. Thus, by drinking ample quantities of water, the colon will become more effective, thus increasing the quantity and supply of fresh blood that can then move throughout the body. And improper blood flow and insulin levels are known migraine triggers.

In short, it is vital that every cell, tissue, and organ be sufficiently hydrated for your body to return to and maintain its natural state of homeostasis. It is only in this state that the chemical toxins that have built up in the body can be properly processed and eliminated. Water is the only substance that can properly hydrate the body; not caffeinated coffees and teas (including herbal teas), carbonated sodas, or sugar-filled fruit drinks. Only water, pure and simple as it is, will keep you healthy and help the body eliminate many of the underlying headache triggers.

Not All Water Is Safe to Drink

Not all water is suitable for drinking. In fact, in cities such as Baltimore, the fecal level in the water supply has been so high in recent years that the government has had to step in and deem the situation a national emergency.

As Robert Milne, M.D., and Blake More note in their *Definitive Guide to Headaches*: " . . . even with a filter, tap water is not the safest to drink, especially if you are headache-prone. . . . With every cup . . . you increase your risk of being exposed to heavy metals and/or chemical toxins, especially . . . during the times the water districts add any of the 700 chemicals available for use."[4]

According to a report published by the Environmental Protection Agency (EPA) in 1993, 819 cities in the United States had exceeded lead levels in their drinking water, and tap water supplied to thirty million people in America contained potentially hazardous levels of lead.[5]

In addition, the EPA offers the following stern warning: "Naturally occurring contaminants also are being found in drinking water. For example, the radioactive gas radon-222 is found in certain types of rock and can get into ground water. People can be exposed to radon in water by drinking it, while showering, or when washing dishes."[6]

Echoing this concern, Drs. Milne and More mention a survey conducted in Illinois, where the drinking water in a small town in the western part of the state had been contaminated by the industrial chemical solvent trichloroethylene (TCE). More than half of the respondents reported severe or frequent headaches caused, in some cases, by merely taking a shower![7]

With this in mind, it is best that headache sufferers not drink water directly from their tap, as natural and chemical toxin buildup in the bloodstream is a definite—though preventable—headache trigger. Thus, drinking purified bottled water or filtered water should be the only option.

How Much Water Is Enough?

There is much written about specific quantities of water that are needed by the body to function properly. Certainly, drinking a single glass of water at lunch or dinner will not do the job. And while the FDA recommends six eight-ounce glasses of water per day, to reap the full health benefits from water one must think in terms of water as therapy and drink copious amounts throughout the entire day.

There are several measures for drinking an appropriate amount of water. For example, Rudolph Ballentine, M.D., suggests that as adults we should optimally consume about eight ounces of water per twenty pounds of body weight. This equals roughly two quarts of water per day. More water is required if it is lost through perspiration from high temperatures or strenuous exercise.[8]

Dr. Batmanghelidj proposes that while adults must consume specific quantities of water, they must also do it at specified times. He asserts the following: "You need water before you sleep because for eight hours you are going to be drying up gradually. . . . Your vascular system expands. You breathe out a lot of water. You manufacture urine. . . . So you are dehydrated. . . . The first thing in the morning, drink two glasses of water."[9]

However, trying to remember specific times and quantities of water to consume can be cumbersome. I personally ascribe to a more liberal method of just drinking water all day and watching my urine color as a gauge for when I need to consume more water. It is generally agreed that adults need at least two quarts of water per day under ideal conditions—and colas, coffee, and iced tea do not count toward this. If you drink water from a bottle throughout the day, after a period of hydration you will find yourself making frequent trips to the restroom to relieve yourself. A continuous flow of water through your body that is continually washing away the toxins in your system and keeping them from building up and triggering headaches is exactly what you want.

If you maintain a constant flow of water through your body, your kidneys will not become overtaxed and forced to concentrate urine in an effort to maintain proper levels of hydration in your body. The sign of proper hydration is urine that is light-colored or clear. When urine is concentrated as a result of dehydration, its color becomes dark. If your urine is dark-colored, it is a sign that you are becoming dehydrated—this happens quickly when consuming caffeinated diuretic beverages like coffee and soda—and it is time for another glass or two of water. I always keep my bottle of spring or filtered water filled and at my side. In this way, I will never forget to drink from it, and I will not be forced to consume chemically treated tap water in whatever location I happen to find myself.

In summary, we have established the undeniable fact that next to air, water is the most vital substance know to man; that keeping the body properly hydrated helps remove toxins from the body while maintaining proper blood flow and organ, muscle, and glandular functions; that it is not necessarily safe to drink tap water; and that drinking water throughout the day, as dictated by urine color, is the best way to maintain proper hydration.

Your body has never felt as light or as clean and unpolluted as it will once it is properly hydrated. And in the process, a large portion of the ongoing headache triggers that have attacked you in the past will be eliminated.

Chapter Five

TOXICITY AND HEADACHE

One of the primary causes of chronic headaches is congestion, or the overconsumption of foods high in pesticides, preservatives, nitrates, refined sugars, fats, caffeinated and alcoholic beverages, environmental toxins, over-the-counter analgesics, and prescription medications. If these toxic elements are not effectively eliminated from the body in a timely matter, they putrefy in the digestive tract and lead to the poisonous toxic buildup in the body that causes headaches.

Overconsumption is directly related to lifestyle choices—the things we choose to eat, drink, and ingest—many of which are predicated on some psycho-physiological "need." It might at first seem odd that in a country such as the United States, where we have ready access to information regarding the latest studies on diet, nutrition, biochemistry, and headaches, and an abundance of fresh fruit, produce, grains, and organic fish and meat at our disposal, millions of Americans each year suffer chronic headaches. Is it because of ignorance or mere laziness that we make such poor dietary choices? Perhaps the answer is grounded in perception and misguided imagery displayed by the media. Consider the following excerpt from a report prepared by Anthony Gallo for the USDA, regarding the $7 billion food manufacturers spent on advertising in 1997: "Most of this advertising focused on highly processed and highly packaged foods. In contrast, the U.S. Department of Agriculture spent $333.3 million on nutrition education, evaluation, and demonstrations. This is approximately what the food industry spent on advertising just for coffee, tea, and cocoa, or for snacks and nuts. . . ."[1]

In the sections that follow, toxicity, constipation, detoxification, and fasting are discussed in terms of their individual and joint roles in the management and ultimate prevention of headaches.

Toxicity and Congestion

Almost anything, if ingested or absorbed into the body in large quantities and not properly eliminated, can become toxic. Most of the toxins our bodies are exposed to derive from chemicals on and in the foods we eat, chemicals in the tap water we drink and wash with, and in pain relievers we take as a matter of habit.

In *The Detox Diet*, Elson Haas, M.D., explains in simple terms how our body is equipped to handle "normal" levels of toxins by neutralizing, transforming, or eliminating them: "The liver helps transform many toxic substances into harmless agents, which the blood carries away to the kidneys; the liver also sends wastes [through] the bile into the intestines, where it is eliminated. We also clear toxins through sweating, . . . excess mucus . . . and skin rashes."[2]

However, it is when toxins overload our system and are not properly or quickly eliminated from it, that we begin poisoning ourselves. The overconsumption of toxic elements with inadequate elimination causes congestion, which leads to toxic buildup, overtaxing the liver, colon, kidneys, and lungs, and hampering their effective functioning. Headaches are a symptom of congestion and toxicity.

One of the primary and most obvious forms of congestion is constipation. Constipation is the stagnant retention of bodily waste products, most of which are toxic chemicals. Transit time for normally functioning individuals is 18 to 24 hours from ingestion of food to elimination through bowel movement. If the body retains the excrement for a longer duration, the feces begin to putrefy, and the chemical toxins reenter the bloodstream, causing headaches (among a host of other health disorders). Is it any wonder that chronic headaches are prevalent in people who are perpetually or chronically constipated? And if you do not pass your bowels more than once per day, you are constipated.

As a consequence of long-standing constipation, the digestive tract, particularly the lower bowels and colon, becomes slack and stagnant with hardened residues clinging to the walls of the colon and filling its many pockets and folds. This results in putrefaction and gas, forming a source of slow poisoning of the whole body. As Oliver Sacks, M.D., confers: "Constipation is, in fact, an integral portion of the migraine."[3]

While a poor diet high in refined sugar and simple carbohydrates and low in fiber is the main cause of constipation, dehydration and overconsumption of coffee and alcohol (both of which are diuretics) also lead to the drying out of the colonic track and thus to constipation, as do stress, anxiety, and low levels of physical activity.

In the previous chapter we discussed the role of water in headaches, and in the next chapter we will discuss the role of diet. Suffice it to say again, however, that without ample quantities of water in the body at all times, constipation and/or headaches are going to result. In addition, a poor diet is sure to induce constipation and/or headaches. A change in eating habits is essential, then, for prevention of headaches in general and toxicity-related headaches in particular. The following dietary guidelines should prevent the onset of constipation and its related headaches.

1. Too little dietary fiber can cause constipation. So, eat more complex carbohydrates. (White bread and pasta do not count!) And, as reported in the *American Journal of Gastroenterology*, oat bran is superior to wheat and corn bran in its ability to lower blood fats.[4] Choosing to do so at breakfast will help you start the day right.

2. Eat more alkaline foods (which have a laxative effect) such as fruits and vegetables, fiber and leafy greens (which aid in stool bulk and softness), and complex carbohydrates, and a smaller proportion of meats and fats.

3. Drink ample amounts of water all day long (to promote toxic elimination) and refrain from or limit your intake of beverages high in sugar, alcohol, and caffeine.

4. Be sure to exercise at least 15 to 30 minutes every day (a brisk walk is great).

5. Be sure to eliminate your bowels when they indicate they are ready—do not hold it in!

Detoxification

Headaches can be triggered by either existing toxins in the colon and intestines or as a result of new toxins entering the system. To be effective, elimination of such headaches must occur on two levels. First, we must purge the system of existing toxins through a program of detoxification and fasting. Second, we must prevent future toxins from entering our systems.

As mentioned in Chapter Four, drinking ample quantities of pure water throughout the day is so vital because it helps clear existing toxins in the body through sweat and urination, while also helping to move new toxins through the system in a timely manner. In his book *Radical*

Healing, Rudolph Ballentine, M.D., has this to say about two of the four primary excretory routes: "The urinary tract and the skin have their problems, too. The full use of them for elimination depends on adequate water intake—as does, to a great extent, the optimal function of the colon. That makes water the key to much of your detoxifying and cleansing efforts."[5]

Dr. Haas concurs, when he writes: "Gastrointestinal function and ecology [are] the core of human health. Imbalances can affect overall well-being. Likewise, the structure and function of the intestines determine total body toxin load and are essential to the process of detoxification. Cleansing and healing the GI tract (especially the colon) provides a base for effective detoxification."[6]

At the top of Dr. Haas's list of signs and symptoms that can be healed by detoxification is headache. Following this, and among some thirty signs and symptoms of toxicity, are tight or stiff neck, circulatory deficits, high blood fats, backaches, irritated eyes, sinus congestion, fever, nervousness, insomnia, anxiety, depression, and constipation. By now we know that all of these are triggers and symptoms of headache.

For a detoxification program to be effective, it must clear congestion by moving toxins from the bowels and otherwise eliminating it through urination and sweat. The colon, intestines, lungs, and liver must all work at optimal efficiency for toxic headache prevention to be effective. For this to happen, toxins must be flushed and excreted from the system. Again, water holds a big place in this process, as do fiber, psyllium supplements, enemas, and the antioxidant vitamins and minerals.

There are many fine detoxification programs available to choose from. While I have personally engaged in several detoxification programs, I do not feel qualified to prescribe one to you. I will, however, suggest you look into the detoxification programs of Dr. Andrew Weil, Dr. Elson Haas, and Dr. Paavo Airola in addition to discussing your constipation or toxic issues with a nutritionist or naturopathic healer for their advice on a program that is best suited to your needs and schedule.

Fasting

Fasting is so important in headache prevention that it should be done periodically throughout the year. How many days you fast will be determined by how toxic and constipated your body has become as a result of what you put into it through your lifestyle choices. Fasting not only gives the digestive system a chance to rest and rejuvenate itself, it also helps move toxins through the system.

Fasting is a time-honored tradition in both healing and religious circles. Rites of passage and initiation often include fasting as an integral part of preparation for transition from one social position to another, as it helps clear the body, mind, and spirit to bring it clean into the new position. As a mechanism of healing, fasting is so entrenched in the lifestyle of many cultures of the world that its importance and effectiveness cannot be contested.

Fasting generally means omitting solid foods from the diet for a period of time. It does not imply starvation, nor does it exclude the ingestion of liquids—which are essential for proper hydration and detoxification. While one-day fasts can be beneficial, many programs advise that at least three days of continuous fasting is necessary to purge the system of poisonous toxins.

There are two primary methods of fasting: water and juice. While water fasts are very effective, some people find them hard to manage. Tasting and filling your body with nothing but plain water for several days can be trying. Fruit juice and vegetable broth fasts seems to be an easier way to go, with as much or more detoxification power.

In his seminal work *How to Get Well*, Dr. Paavo Airola notes that by the early 1970s Dr. Otto H. F. Buchinger had supervised more than 80,000 raw-juice fasts! "In his experience," Dr. Airola explains, "fasting on the fresh raw juices of fruits and vegetable broth and herbal teas results in much faster recovery from disease and more effective cleansing and rejuvenation of the tissues than does the traditional water fast."[7]

Regarding the water-versus-juice-fasting dichotomy, Dr. Haas's findings are in agreement with those of Dr. Airola and Dr. Buchinger: "Fresh juices are easily assimilated and require minimum digestion, while still supplying many nutrients and stimulating our body to clear wastes. It is also safer than water fasting as it supports the body nutritionally while cleansing and hence maintains bodily energy levels, producing better detoxification and a quicker recovery."[8]

Most juice fasts require that the juice you consume be made fresh daily with only organic fruit or vegetables. You can do it yourself with a juicer or purchase the juices or broths from a health food store or farmers' market. It is vital that you not fast with fruits or vegetables bought from your local chain food superstore, as these most likely contain chemical toxins and pesticides that will only add to your headache problem.

The aim of fasting is to engage body detoxification. The main way these toxins are expelled or purged from the body is through the digestive and eliminative (gastrointestinal) system. However, during fasting toxins in the digestive and elimination tracts have no way of leaving the body since liquids alone do not excite the defecation reflex. You see, bowel movements are activated by muscle contractions in the intestines caused by the filled rectum, and since fasting is not causing ample pressure in that area, an enema is necessary. The enema fills the rectum with water and causes enough pressure to activate the muscle contraction necessary to force elimination of waste products in the bowels.

Many fine fasting programs are available. I have personally participated in a 72-hour water-only qigong-energy fast as well as fruit juice fasts and cabbage-based soup fasts and experienced different results from each of them. Again, while I cannot prescribe a fast for you personally, I do recommend that you speak with your nutritionist or naturopathic healer about it.

In summary, toxic headaches are triggered by congestion or constipation of putrefied food and toxic chemicals in the system as a result of insufficient elimination. Ample water intake every day as well as exercise and eating a diet high in fiber, complex carbohydrates, and high-alkaline foods and low in sugar, saturated fats, and caffeine are simple ways of keeping "regular" and preventing toxic buildup in the body. In addition, it is necessary at least once per year to engage in a full detox program and fast to help purge the system—especially if lifestyle choices have not allowed a proper diet to be followed as a matter of habit.

Chapter Six

DIET AND HEADACHE

Do you wake up in the morning tired, with only enough time to devour a plain bagel and cup of coffee? For lunch, do you settle for a quick cold-cut sandwich on a roll made of bleached white flour and a soft drink? For dinner do you enjoy a nice Italian dinner, red wine, coffee, and dessert? If you answered yes to one or all of these questions and suffer chronic headaches, chances are that food sensitivities may be the culprit.

There are a number of ways in which the food and beverages we consume contribute to and/or directly cause headaches. As discussed in the previous chapter, simple food allergies or sensitivities and chemical toxins play a major role in headaches. Low blood sugar and high levels of fat in the blood are also notorious headache triggers. In recent years a number of scientific studies have shown a direct correlation between low levels of serotonin in the blood and headaches; and the chemical tyramine, which is found in many foods, and has been found to decrease serotonin levels.

In the sections below, we'll see what foods are known to trigger headaches in sufferers prone to food sensitivities. We'll also look at how low blood sugar and high blood fat contribute to headaches, and we'll learn how to balance them through diet. And we'll see just how foods we eat can decrease serotonin and why low levels of this neurotransmitter causes headaches. Following this will be nutritional and dietary guidelines for establishing a responsible eating regime and habits and explain which vitamins and minerals are important in headache prevention.

Food Sensitivities

Many chronic migraine sufferers know that eating certain foods can trigger their headaches. This is due to a number of reasons: Often the individual has an allergy or sensitivity to the particular food; the food may be causing a rise or decline in blood sugar or blood fat; or it could be that chemical preservatives are leaving a toxic residue in the body. Sometimes it is a food's inherent stimulant or depressant attributes or its ability to decrease levels of serotonin.

Among the foods reported time and again by headache sufferers to trigger their headaches are alcohol (red wine), caffeinated beverages (coffee, tea, soda), dairy products (ice cream, milk), Aspartame (NutraSweet, Equal), MSG, sodium nitrates, processed and preserved meats (beef jerky, cold cuts), certain fruits (unripe bananas, unripe apples, papayas, avocados, dried fruits), foods containing the amino acid tyramine (nuts, aged cheese, pickled foods), milk chocolate, raw onions, sauerkraut, and some beans (lentils and lima beans).

Alcohol has been causing headaches since the first drink was poured. Aside from your basic hangover resulting from overconsumption of this adult beverage, even small amounts of alcohol can trigger headaches in a number of ways. For starters, alcohol is a diuretic, and we already know that dehydration causes headaches. Alcohol is also a vasodilator, which means it not only contributes to rebound headaches but also hinders the liver's ability to metabolize carbohydrates. When carbohydrates are not properly broken down or burned off through exercise, your body changes their excess sugars to glucose, which raises blood sugar levels, activating the release of insulin. If there is too much alcohol in the bloodstream, too much insulin will be released and cause blood sugar levels to fall too low, and a hypoglycemic headache will result. What's more, even when alcohol is eliminated from the body through sweating, urine, and feces, it leaves a fat byproduct in its wake, which not only causes toxicity but also raises blood fat levels, both of which cause headaches. Moreover, the sulfites in red wine are infamous triggers for many migraine sufferers. For chronic headache sufferers, then, it is best to either abstain from alcohol completely or limit intake to only a few times per year.

Among the most notorious headache-inducing chemicals in our everyday diet is caffeine. Coffee, black or green tea, most soft drinks, cocoa, and many over-the-counter medications (e.g., Excedrin, cough syrups) are the main culprits. On average, we Americans consume over ten pounds of this legal, addictive stimulant each year in the form of coffee alone.

Like most food sensitivities, caffeine can trigger headaches in a number of ways: toxic pesticides and other chemicals used in growing coffee; the natural acids and oils contained in coffee, tea, and cocoa; and caffeine's natural stimulant property, which triggers the rebound headache effect. Moreover, like alcohol, caffeine is a natural diuretic and leads to dehydration. It also causes breathing difficulties and insomnia, stress and anxiety, imbalances in blood sugar and cholesterol levels, dilation and constriction of blood vessels, and depletion of vitamins and minerals such as potassium, magnesium, essential B vitamins, thiamine, and vitamin C. Each one of these individually is a known headache trigger. Together they wreak havoc on the body's ability to maintain homeostasis and bring on any combination of "mixed" headaches (migraine, muscle-contraction, toxic, rebound, sensitivity).

If you think you're safe drinking decaffeinated coffee, think again. Not only do most decaffeinated brands still contain 7 percent caffeine content, but methylene chloride, the main chemical used in the decaffeination process, is toxic to the system. If you simply love coffee so much that you just can't live without it, decaf is your best bet as long as it has been decaffeinated using what is known as the Swiss water process, and the beans themselves are certified organic.

Milk is another no-no when it comes to headaches. Despite huge advertising campaigns and governmental backing espousing ideas to the contrary, all my research indicates that animal milk is unfit for human consumption. It contains high levels of pathogenic bacteria, chemicals, drugs, pesticide residues, hormones, antibiotics, and other harmful and toxic chemicals. Moreover, milk-based products, such as cheese and ice cream, are known headache triggers. If it is unnatural for animals to feed on their mother's own milk after the period of weaning, it just doesn't make sense for humans to consume it at all.

However, calcium deficiency and the possible onset of osteoporosis are issues for women, especially after menopause. For this, I recommend taking calcium carbonate with meals—it's found in antacid products such as Tums and Rolaids. One tablet with each meal should suffice. If you'd prefer supplements, I recommend Solgar's Calcium Magnesium Plus Boron. However, if you're not concerned about calcium but rather enjoy the taste and consistency of milk, I recommend that you try organic soy milk or rice milk. They do the job with cereal and decaf, contain no chemical additives or mucus-forming properties, and simply taste great!

Blood Sugar and Blood Fat

Low blood sugar, high blood sugar, and high blood fat have been proven in hundreds of clinical studies to trigger headaches (among a host of other ailments and diseases). Since increases and decreases in levels of blood sugar and fat result from our dietary choices, we can choose to avoid these triggers and their resultant headaches. With increased blood sugars and fats, the culprit is often a diet constructed around refined sugar (sucrose), animal and hydrogenated fats, simple carbohydrates, caffeinated and alcoholic beverages, along with dehydration and the skipping of meals.

Sugar in the body is not always bad and is actually necessary, as long as the sugar is of the right kind. You see, the human body is biologically set up for the effective breakdown and use of fructose, the natural sugar found in fruits and vegetables. During the digestive process, the body breaks fructose down and turns it into glucose or blood sugar, our primary source of energy. An abundance of glucose also triggers the release of insulin, which not only stabilizes blood sugar levels but also metabolizes fat in the body.

Problems arise for the chronic headache sufferer when sucrose, or refined sugar, enters the bloodstream. While fructose is nature's natural sugar and glucose is the body's broken-down version for energy use, sucrose is an unnatural hybrid of the two natural forms of sugar, which is extremely difficult for the body to metabolize. This leads to toxic buildup in the bloodstream and causes blood sugar levels to rise and then fall from the release of too much insulin, thus creating both toxic and rebound headaches.

There is a direct correlation between sugar levels in the body and blood fat levels, and both can cause headaches, independent of the other. In his book *Maximum Energy*, Ted Broer discusses the role of fiber not only in stabilizing blood sugars but in its ability to reduce blood fats: "Fiber has the unique ability to bond with dietary fats and cholesterol . . . and to transform them into a complex that cannot be absorbed in the digestive tract. . . . The fat and cholesterol . . . are eliminated relatively quickly with defecation, thus lowering total levels of dietary fat and cholesterol in the blood."[1]

The best way to prevent headaches brought on as a result of "bad" blood sugar levels and high levels of cholesterol and triglycerides in the bloodstream is a diet rich in whole grains, complex carbohydrates, vegetables, fruits, proteins, and water, and abstinence from beverages high in caffeine and alcohol.

Serotonin, Tyramine, Tryptophan, and the B Vitamins

One of the main chemical triggers of migraine headaches is a low level of serotonin in the body. Serotonin is a neurotransmitter that carries information from nerve ends to different parts of the body, where it is detected by special receptors and causes a wide range of physiological and psychological reactions.

Serotonin also plays the lead role in controlling depression, anxiety, eating and sleeping patterns, inhibiting pain, and preventing blood vessels from dilating too much. When serotonin levels are low, blood vessels dilate, causing headaches; sleep is disrupted, causing headaches; depression sets in, leading to inactivity and eating disorders, which cause headaches; and pain is able to move easily and powerfully among the nerve endings.

Numerous scientific studies and clinical trials have shown a clear relationship between low levels of serotonin and headache. Test subjects of one such study, when injected with a drug that depletes serotonin, got headaches. Likewise, when they were injected with serotonin, the headaches went away.[2]

A number of things can cause serotonin levels to drop, including a lack of vitamin B_6 and the amino acid tryptophan, and ingestion of high levels of tyramine. All of these are directly linked to diet. Essential B vitamins and tryptophan are found in many fruits, vegetables, grains, and legumes, and a lack of essential vitamins and minerals in the body reflects poor eating habits. Caffeine is also known to deplete B vitamins. Turkey is a good source of tryptophan, which increases the production of serotonin. This in part explains why you feel so tired after Thanksgiving dinner.

Tyramine is a vasoactive amino acid found in foods and is thought to dilate blood vessels. Foods that contain tyramine (such as nuts, cheese, pickled foods) may cause headaches in migraineurs by facilitating a chain reaction, which results in vasoconstriction followed by rebound dilation of the cranial vessels.

Maintaining proper elevated levels of serotonin is therefore vital to chronic headache sufferers in general and migraineurs in particular. This is as easy (or as difficult) as eating a diet low in tyramine-containing foods and high in complex carbohydrates, legumes, seeds, and grains with moderate protein intake. These foods elevate tryptophan levels in the body, which are essential for the production of serotonin.

General Nutrition Guidelines

Overconsumption of a high-fat meal accompanied by alcohol and followed by coffee and dessert is a sure way of bringing on a headache in a timely manner. Oxygen deprivation, high blood sugar followed by hypoglycemia, high blood fat, toxins, and caffeine—all of these overtax the body, with the resultant headache a clear sign that such overindulgence should be avoided in the future.

For headache sufferers, knowing what, when, and how to eat is just as important as knowing what to avoid eating. And good nutrition plays a critical role in headache prevention. While I do not present specific meal schedules and diet plans here, I do offer general dietary guidelines that will help manage and prevent diet-related headaches from occurring.

Dietary fiber is so important in headache prevention that it should be an essential part of your food intake. Fiber keeps the bowels functioning properly for efficient elimination, stabilizes blood sugar levels, and clears fats from the bloodstream. The American Dietetic Association and the American Cancer Society have recommended that we consume from twenty-five to thirty grams of fiber daily, which is abundant in plant products such as fruits, grains, and vegetables.

There are two forms of fiber: soluble and insoluble. Soluble fiber such as pectin (found in most fruits) and oat bran dissolves easily in water so it can be absorbed in the intestine and circulate in the bloodstream. Soluble fiber in the blood has the ability to attach itself to blood fats and create a complex that will remove these fats from the blood system, thus lowering cholesterol.

Insoluble fiber (found in wheat bran, psyllium seed, and citrus membranes) absorbs in water also, but it is not absorbed in the intestine. It remains there and forms the majority of bulk necessary to "sweep" bodily wastes through the intestine and out of the body. Without fiber, food waste and bodily processes move very slowly through the colon (if at all); an abnormally slow-moving mass can putrefy or rot right in the body.[3]

In addition to fiber, seeds and grains are gold mines of minerals, especially calcium, phosphorus, magnesium, and iron. They contain most of the vitamins, particularly vitamins A and E and the B vitamins. They are nature's best source of unsaturated fatty acids and lecithin, and they're excellent sources of protein.

Vitamins and minerals are also important in headache prevention. For example:

✦ Vitamin A helps the development of cells, the growth of bones and teeth, and the maintenance of skin and glands, while decreasing levels of fat in the blood, boosting immunity, and improving night vision. Beta-carotene converts into vitamin A. Good sources include eggs, leafy green vegetables, broccoli, carrots, and peaches.

✦ Vitamin B_2 (riboflavin) is essential for proper functioning of vitamins B_6 and B_3, and it helps you metabolize carbohydrates, fats, and proteins while also helping to convert tryptophan to niacin. Good sources include organ meat, green leafy vegetables, enriched cereal, bread, and eggs.

✦ Vitamin B_3 (niacin) helps lower blood fat by helping to process fat and produce sugar. It is instrumental in the removal of waste from the tissues and the reduction of blood cholesterol. Good sources of vitamin B_3 include meat and eggs. Be sure to stay away from niacin/B_3 supplements, though, as they may cause liver damage.

✦ Vitamin B_5 (pantothenic acid) is essential for protein synthesis and for healing of tissues. It also acts as a stress reducer when combined with other vitamins, such as C. Good sources include eggs, whole grain foods, beans, and most vegetables.

✦ Vitamin B_6 (pyridoxine) helps produce serotonin from tryptophan, helps metabolize fats, produces antibodies, and expedites the conversion of glycogen to glucose. It also helps the body process proteins and carbohydrates, aids in production of blood cells, and strengthens the nervous system. Natural sources of vitamin B_6 include poultry, fish, eggs, spinach, and potatoes.

✦ Vitamin B_{12} is essential for the normal functioning of the cells, nervous system, and gastrointestinal tract. Ample amounts of this vitamin are found in beef, chicken, and fish.

✦ Vitamin C (ascorbic acid) works as an antioxidant to counter free radicals. It is also necessary for the production of serotonin. Vitamin C also strengthens blood vessels, protects the body from bacterial toxins, helps metabolize tyrosine and trypto-phan, and works as an antihistamine. Most people get more than the recommended daily allowance by eating plenty of fruit, broccoli, peppers, and leafy green vegetables.

✦ Vitamin E is strong in antioxidant properties; it protects pitu-itary, adrenal, and sex hormones; it increases the rate at which new blood vessels develop around damaged areas; and it helps to normalize blood viscosity. Good sources include meat, nuts, vegetable oil, and leafy green vegetables.

✦ Chromium stimulates the enzymes involved in glucose metabo-lism, it increases the effectiveness of insulin, and it stimulates the synthesis of fatty acids. As such, it is believed to help reduce the risk of diabetes. Good sources include whole grain cereal, meats, corn oil, and clams.

✦ Potassium stimulates nerve impulses, acts with sodium to regu-late fluids and stimulate the kidneys, and helps convert glucose to glycogen. Recent studies have indicated that potassium is also helpful in reducing blood pressure and reducing the risks of hy-pertension. A good source of potassium is bananas, and as long as they are ripe they should not affect migraineurs.

✦ Selenium is an important antioxidant for chemical detoxification. Good sources include grains, meat, onions, and some vegetables (depending on the selenium content in the soil).

✦ Zinc is necessary for absorption of the B-complex vitamins. It is a component of insulin and is a constituent of more than twenty-five enzymes involved in digestion and metabolism. In addition to zinc supplements, kelp is a good natural source of this mineral.

With regard to cooking oil, only use oils that are neither hydrogenated nor partially hydrogenated. The best type of oil to use is cold-pressed virgin olive oil or canola oil, as these contain safe levels of mono-unsaturated fat. Baking, steaming, or grilling are also healthful options that require no oil at all.

When and How to Eat

Now that we know what not to consume and what to include in our diets, let's look at when and how to eat. On a fundamental level, we need to eat to live and lack of adequate blood sugar—hypoglycemia—is a known cause of headaches. Along with undereating, overeating also causes headaches. It is therefore essential that the migraineur or headache sufferer eat frequent smaller meals to prevent headaches due to overconsumption of food and imbalances in blood sugar levels. I recommend eating one-third-sized portions every 3 hours in an effort to keep energy levels high and blood sugar and serotonin levels stabilized.

It is also important to chew your food properly and completely before swallowing, as this creates sufficient levels of saliva to aid in enzyme breakdown and digestion. Eating more slowly also decreases the amount of food one consumes and makes the meal itself more relaxing and enjoyable.

While it is essential to drink plenty of pure water throughout the day, it is inadvisable to consume too much liquid during meals. Liquids other than saliva dilute the stomach fluids necessary for proper metabolism and digestion of the food you eat.

As you can see, there are numerous headache triggers associated with diet, body chemicals, and headaches—and every one of them is related to lifestyle choices. Follow a healthy eating program high in fruits, vegetables, and complex carbohydrates, and avoid caffeine, refined sugar, simple carbohydrates, tyramine-containing foods, and alcohol. Eat frequently, chew your food well, and don't drink too much during meal time. Feed your body well, and you'll be rewarded with well-being as the headache triggers directly linked with diet are stricken from your life.

Chapter Seven

EXERCISE AND HEADACHE

Engaging in the right type and level of exercise for at least 20 minutes at a time several days per week is a powerful tool in preventing headaches. In one activity we are able to increase blood flow, decrease blood sugars and fats, burn calories, reduce adipose tissue, increase oxygen flow to the brain, increase our resting metabolism, loosen the musculoskeletal system, and detoxify the body while improving digestion and eliminative functions. Without a doubt, exercise is an essential part of the integrated mind/body approach to headache prevention.

In this chapter, we'll look at how exercise can help prevent headaches and the processes involved therein. We'll also take a look at which exercises are best for headache sufferers, learn some methods of correcting somatic imbalances, and see why rest and sleep are just as important to headache prevention as exercise itself.

The Healing Power of Exercise

The utilization of stored energy is what propels the human body and gives it the fuel necessary to do such basic things as stand, bend, and lift objects. We derive this energy mainly from the complex carbohydrates we eat, which are stored in the body as sugars and fats.

Energy is released in the body through the process of respiration. During any physical activity we breathe in air. Oxygen from that breath moves into the bloodstream where it is transported to the organs and utilized to burn the stored sugar and fat "fuel." The waste product of this process is carbon dioxide, and this passes back into the bloodstream, back into the lungs, and then is removed from the body on exhale. The greater the duration and higher the intensity of physical exercise, the greater the amount of oxygen is taken into the body and moved into the bloodstream, and the more carbon dioxide waste is expelled from the body.

There are basically two types of exercise, or methods of utilizing stored sugars and fat: anaerobic and aerobic. Anaerobic exercise does not require oxygen, instead burning glucose (derived from carbohydrates) from the muscle's store of sugar reserves (glycogen). However, these reserves are quickly depleted and the body must then draw its energy from stored body fat and blood fat. This requires oxygen, and so this type of exercise is called aerobic. Since aerobic exercise utilizes oxygen, stored glucose, and fat, it is able to burn fat calories, decrease the resting heart rate, increase oxygen flow to the brain, and ease stress and muscle tension by releasing beta-endorphins, the body's natural pain reliever. Thus, both anaerobic and aerobic exercises contribute greatly to our headache prevention program.

Our aim in preventing headaches is to return the body to its natural balanced state of homeostasis. Both anaerobic and aerobic exercises contribute to this by increasing both blood flow and oxygen flow, which help stabilize blood vessels (by supplying a steady supply of oxygen to the brain) and normalize blood sugars and blood fats (by utilizing them for energy). And we know that dilating and constricting blood vessels and high levels of fats and sugars in the bloodstream are direct causes of headaches.

Regular exercise is also a powerful tool in our efforts toward detoxification. Since prolonged physical activity activates the sweat glands, it enables elimination of wastes and toxins through the skin. Since exercise utilizes fats and sugars for energy, it burns calories and eliminates toxins from our system. Toxins are also released through the breath and bowel functions, and both are improved through exercise.

The Two Best Exercises

There are so many different types of exercises available and so many places to do them, that to begin a program can seem daunting, especially if a sedentary lifestyle has been the norm.

The thrust of the program put forth in this book is headache prevention by means of self-direction. It is not necessary to join a gym or to purchase a treadmill in order to prevent headaches through exercise; indeed, immediately joining an aerobics class or churning out miles on a treadmill can actually cause headaches if you are not currently "in shape." As with any effort that involves changing lifestyle patterns and outlooks, it is best to start slowly, enjoy yourself, and build to more challenging activities as your body and interests support them.

I don't personally enjoy lifting weights, jogging, or doing aerobics. However, I do train in the martial arts and engage in a regular program of qigong standing and brisk walking as mind/body exercises. Since our headache program incorporates an integrated mind/body theme, this must be an essential component of the physical activity you choose as exercise. In this way, in addition to burning calories, increasing oxygen flow, and stabilizing blood fats and sugars, you will also develop a mind/body center that will help focus your thoughts, emotions, and spirit, thus helping to reduce the stress and anxiety that trigger headaches.

BRISK WALKING

If done correctly, brisk walking can be one of the safest and most beneficial and enjoyable of exercises. Walking is an aerobic activity, but since it is low-impact there is little wear and tear on the joints and little (if any) triggering of headaches from the jarring action of the body experienced in high-impact aerobic exercise or jogging. Although it is a simple activity, walking actually utilizes most of the muscles of the body to propel you forward and keep you on balance while increasing respiration, heart and lung function, blood and oxygen flow, the "burning off" of blood sugars and fats, and removal of toxins and other wastes through sweat and improved eliminative functions.

In her detailed book *Walk Yourself Well*, walking guru Sherry Brourman says this about the activity: "Walking 30 minutes a day can raise HDL levels, improve circulation and heart function, help with weight reduction and maintenance, reduce stress and promote relaxation, [and] increase muscle strength and endurance."[1]

Many of the triggers that attack headache sufferers can be reduced or eliminated simply by walking. To go for a walk, all you need is time and a sidewalk, road, or trail—no special place, though it is preferable to walk in a park as opposed to a busy city sidewalk.

Though walking in and of itself is a common activity, few of us do it properly. In fact, casual walking will do little for headache prevention. You must look to walking as a mind/body activity, wherein your mind is clear, emotions calm, respiration slow and steady, body properly aligned and relaxed, and your steps even and balanced. If you are able to integrate each of these components while briskly walking for at least

20 minutes a day, then your walks can be considered a microcosm of the integrated mind/body approach to headache prevention. If you are interested in learning more about the health, spiritual, and meditative benefits walking can provide, I recommend the book *Warrior Walking* by Josh Holzer.[2]

QIGONG STANDING

Qigong is an ancient Chinese mind/body discipline that seeks to establish a healthy body by developing the so-called three treasures and three regulations.

The three treasures are known as *jing* (essence), *qi* (vital energy), and *shen* (spirit). *Jing* is simply the body's energy that is derived from glycogen and turned into glucose and used to propel the body during any physical activity. *Qi* has many meanings, many of which are esoteric and difficult to comprehend in Western terms. However, all of these meanings and definitions involve the coordination of breath or respiration with concentration. *Shen* encompasses the many functions of the mind. Qigong is primarily concerned with the *yi* functions (focus, intention, and thought), as it is the intention that leads the breath to develop energy to power the body and make us healthy.

Qigong practice greatly supports our efforts at establishing homeostasis by nurturing the "three treasures" which in turn normalize the "three regulations," which are the body, the respiration, and the mind. When all three are centered or regulated, then a healthy state of being can be achieved.

I have personally been studying various forms of qigong in the United States and Asia for more than fifteen years. I have found that while there are hundreds of qigong practices, they all focus on the three treasures and three regulations. For the headache sufferer—especially those with chronic musculoskeletal headache triggers—the simpler the system, the better. Thus, I have chosen to describe here the method known as *zhanzhuang*, or simply the "standing pole" qigong. It requires only enough space to stand still and will not distract the mind by requiring you to remember specific sequences of movement. While the complete *zhanzhuang* "health" (as opposed to martial art) practice engages eight or more postures, only one is needed here.

In a nutshell, this practice is as easy as standing with your legs shoulder width apart with the knees bent only 1 to 2 inches, with both arms bent at the elbow 90 degrees with forearms parallel with the ground and palms facing down. Try to visualize that your forearms and palms are floating on water. Once the posture is assumed, quiet the mind by not stressing over distracting thoughts that may come—simply allow them to go freely without judgment. Next, regulate respiration by quietly breathing in and out at a steady relaxed pace. Now enjoy yourself for the next 20 minutes. You'll be surprised to find how difficult merely standing still can be, but you'll derive numerous benefits as a result.

There are a number of great books available on the *zhanzhuang* or standing pole qigong exercises by such notable masters Lam Kam Chuan, Paul Dong, and Wang Xuanjie. To explain further the inherent benefits of this mind/body exercise, I would like to quote from the book *Traditional Chinese Therapeutic Exercises—Standing Pole*, by Wang Xuanjie and J. P. C. Moffett: "Standing pole is an exercise of the whole body. As the outer form of the body is not moved, all the internal organs settle, while all metabolic functions increase. This develops movement within non-movement, that is, . . . simultaneously providing rest and exercise . . . and encouraging development of the body's innate strengths and abilities in a natural way."[3]

You see, while it appears as if you are doing nothing at all, in actuality the body is engaged in a process of physical activity. While quieting the mind and regulating respiration we are reducing stress, relaxing the cerebral cortex, and rejuvenating the central nervous system—all essential to preventing headaches. Moreover, we are also working the muscles by virtue of maintaining a posture wherein the knees and elbows are bent, the arms are raised, and this must be held steady without release until the end of the session. Thus, we are elevating our heart rate without overtaxing the heart, improving the circulation of blood and oxygen throughout the body, and increasing metabolic functions while releasing toxins and tension from the body.

Correcting Somatic Imbalances

We already know that tension-type headaches are caused by muscle contractions and pinched nerves, which not only decrease blood flow and oxygen flow in the body, but also cause structural misalignment and nerve-ending irritation.

A sore neck and tense shoulders are common among those who spend hours a day seated at desks or behind the wheels of vehicles, and in those who, regardless of vocation, harbor stress and anxiety in their bodies. This causes not only nerve pain but muscle contractions in the base of the skull, which can cause severe head pain, which can then trigger a migraine headache. It is therefore important that we keep the body relaxed and supple through a program of general stretching with specific focus given to the neck, shoulders, spine, and hips. These are the areas that are most affected by poor posture and unreleased stresses and tensions, thus triggering muscle-contraction or tension-type headaches in those who are susceptible to them.

There are a number of bodywork therapy programs and methods available. I personally utilize exercises from Western sports science, Eastern qigong, liangong, and yoga, as well as the Feldenkrais Method and the Alexander Technique. Each of these bodywork therapy systems is easy to perform and works wonders on specific body parts. Since each of these somatic (or body) exercises is based on relaxation and not exertion, it is very difficult to injure yourself doing them. Thus, reading some books or viewing videos on them is generally enough to get you started. While it is of course necessary to enroll in a class to fully learn each of these disciplines, prolonged class attendance is not necessary for our purpose here, which is simply the prevention of muscle-contraction headaches.

GENERAL STRETCHING GUIDELINES

A basic first step in preventing muscle-contraction headaches (as well as avoiding injury while exercising) is loosening the muscles of the body, thereby releasing chronic strain and tension while improving overall blood flow.

While there are hundreds of stretches and thousands of programs and books available on them, they generally fall into the categories of progressive relaxation stretches (those which allow the muscle to relax while held in a fixed position), progressive resistance stretches (those which force relaxation through isometrically fatiguing the muscle group), and ballistic stretches (those which use bouncing to force flexibility). For the purposes of headache prevention, it is not necessary to achieve the great flexibility required of some sports. Rather, it is important only to relax, become supple, and achieve a general sense of "feeling good." Therefore, do not strain or worry while stretching, just relax and let the stretch happen of its own accord. It is best, then, to engage in progressive relaxation with full range of muscle-joint motion.

Before stretching the muscle you must first loosen the joints, of which there are two types: hinge and ball-and-socket. Hinge joints are those that move back and forth, like your fingers and knees. Ball-and-socket joints are those that rotate, like your elbows and hips.

Begin by slowly bending and/or rotating every joint from your toes to your neck, in order and one at a time. A count of five to ten bends or rotations per joint in each direction is sufficient to get things properly lubricated and loosened, and if you methodically work your way from the bottom up you will not inadvertently skip anything. The sequence would then be: toes, ankles, knees, hips, fingers, wrists, elbows, shoulders, neck, and jaw.

Once the joints are supple you can move on to the muscles, beginning again from the feet and working your way up to the neck. Stretches can be done seated on the floor, on a chair, or while standing. Whether you choose to stand or sit while stretching, it is important to remain calm, breathe steadily, and keep all muscles that are not being stretched relaxed. In other words, only the muscle being worked should feel tension and release. Again, stretching the muscles in the following order should make things easy while not skipping anything: calfs, quadriceps, thighs, groin, hips and buttocks, forearm, triceps, deltoids, shoulders, and neck.

EXERCISING THE NECK AND SHOULDERS

The following somatic exercises are derived from the Chinese health system known as liangong, which is a set of eighteen exercises specific for keeping the neck, shoulders, waist, and legs fit, supple, and in proper musculoskeletal alignment.[4] These exercises do much to help prevent headaches by initiating muscle contraction which detoxifies stagnant blood stored in tight muscles and those in spasm, improves the mobility of the joints, loosens soft tissue adhesions, realigns the spine, and otherwise balances the structural system, while increasing overall blood and oxygen flow.

1. Stand with feet slightly wider than shoulder width, with hands open and palms facing out held a few inches from the face. Thumbs and index finger should be pointing toward each other.

2. Close your hands and turn your head to your left while separating your arms until your forearms are at a 90-degree angle to your biceps. Shoulders should rotate backward during the motion to open the chest area.

3. Return to the starting position and repeat on the opposite side.

4. Be sure to move slowly, while keeping respiration steady and your shoulders down. Repeat the left/right sequence ten times.

5. After the last repetition, return head and arms to forward facing position, clench both fists, and lower your elbows until your fists are aligned with your shoulders. This is the next starting position.

6. Open the fists while reaching and stretching both arms up above your head, with palms facing forward, head raised, and eyes looking at the fingers of the right hand. While reaching upward it is important to push out the chest and suck in the abdomen slightly.

7. Return to the new starting position and repeat the upward arm stretch, this time with the eyes looking at the fingers of the right hand.

8. Be sure to move slowly and steadily and do not hold your breath. Repeat the left/right sequence ten times.

STRETCHING THE NECK AND SHOULDERS

The following neck flexion positions will do much to stretch the neck and shoulder muscles, thus decreasing stiffness and chances of occipital headache as a result of muscle contraction of shoulders and neck.

1. Sit with head forward and back straight on a chair or other stable surface, being certain to keep the spine erect.

2. Slowly allow your head to drop forward.

3. Firmly clasp your hands behind your head, just above your neck, being sure not to squeeze your head or grasp your neck.

4. Gently and slowly pull your head toward your chest until you feel a nice, comfortable stretch.

5. Breathe slowly and hold for 30 seconds.

6. Release your grip and slowly return your head to its upright position.

7. Next, while keeping your shoulders and hips aligned, turn your head and look to your right.

8. Place your right hand on the back of the top of your head and gently pull your head down so that your chin touches your armpit.

9. Relax, breathe easily, and hold for 30 seconds.

10. Release your grip and slowly return your head to its upright position.

11. Repeat steps seven through ten on your left side.

Restorative Rest and Sleep

Mathematically, it would seem that the average person spends nearly one-third of his life asleep—or at least in bed. However, statistics show that sleep disorders are among the nation's most common health problems, affecting up to seventy million people. For those suffering chronic headaches, sleep is often something they get too much of or too little of. Either extreme is a bad thing.

Sleep deprivation is a sure trigger of headaches, and anxiety, stress, poor digestion, and low levels of serotonin lead to poor sleeping patterns. Proper, sound sleep happens in distinct stages, and these stages regulate the deep-tissue healing of our muscles, relax the nervous systems, regulate hormones, and help reestablish homeostasis.

Improper restorative rest after exercise or long weeks of stress-laden work, general insomnia, or the inability to sleep straight through the night do much to trigger both migraine headaches and muscle-contraction headaches. If you do get a sound sleep but also experience headaches on waking, it may be caused by either lack of oxygen to the brain or from poor sleep posture, which puts pressure on nerves and stunts blood flow in the body during the evening hours—and this, we know, can cause headaches.

Robert Milne, M.D., and Blake More have this to say about rest and headache: "Adequate rest is essential to any health-related regimen, particularly since too little of it makes you a prime candidate for headaches. The brain chemicals that govern sleeping and waking cycles are the same ones that have been linked to headaches: serotonin and norepinephrine."[5] The doctors go on to further say that erratic sleeping patterns or missed sleep lead to an imbalance of serotonin and norepinephrine. Moreover, they note that many sleep disturbances are in fact caused by a dysfunctional digestive system and liver detoxification pathways.

Knowing this now partially explains why I got so many headaches in college: eating nitrate-heavy fast foods, staying up all night to study and write papers, taking successions of cat naps between classes to make up for the lack of sleep, and the stiff neck and cramped shoulders resulting from sleeping with arms and head resting on the library study tables.

Getting a sound sleep and doing so in a posture that will neither cramp the muscles nor constrict air supply is vital to preventing headaches. The best position to sleep in is lying on your back with arms by their respective sides, head and neck straight and slightly elevated. Another good posture is the fetal position, as long as the arms are kept in front of the body and not shoved under the pillow or raised above the head. There are several ergonomic pillows available today that make finding a comfortable yet proper sleeping posture easy.

For those of you who suffer from insomnia or sleep apnea, I would like to offer the following three-step suggestion. First, stay away from caffeinated beverages after six o'clock in the evening (or at any time!). Second, place a notepad next to your bed and when your mind starts racing with things that need to get done, or people that need to be called, simply write it down and let it go until the morning. Lying awake in bed at night will in no way help these things get done; it only amplifies stress and anxiety and prevents sleep. Third, try the following progressive relaxation technique to induce a deep state of calm and relaxation that should allow you to drift off to sleep in a short time while allowing your body and nervous system to rejuvenate itself:

1. Lie on your back with arms at your sides and slowly inhale and exhale with no sound.

2. Do cyclical breathing, with a 4-second count for a full inhalation and an 8-second count for a full exhalation. Do at least ten repetitions; more if necessary.

3. Once your respiration is calm and even, return to normal breathing and begin progressively relaxing every part of your body by mentally focusing on that area, calmly willing it to relax and retaining your intention there until the part begins to tingle.

4. Begin by relaxing the toes of the left leg, one at a time. Then move on to the sole of the foot, the ankle, the calf, and so on until you reach the hips. Then do the same with the right leg.

5. Move progressively up to the buttocks, hips, back, arms, chest, shoulders, neck, and face.

This process induces such a deep state of relaxation that most people fall asleep before reaching their arms. Give it a try and see how it goes. And if you find it difficult at first, don't stress out—it's only a relaxation technique. Let your thoughts go and enjoy the process, and perhaps sooner than later it will take hold and you will begin enjoying the deep, full sleep that may have been missing from your life for many years.

If your wakeful night is the result of obstructed breathing, then oxygen deprivation will double your chances of a morning headache. I suggest trying one or more of the many anti-snore devices on the market, such as Nozovent, Noiselezz, or SomnoGuard.

Sweet dreams!

Chapter 8

STRESS AND HEADACHE

Stress is one of the leading causes of illness in the United States, and one of the main triggers of headaches. According to Oliver Sacks, M.D., "nearly two-thirds of ailments seen in doctors' offices are commonly thought to be stress-induced or related to stress in some way."[1]

The effects of stress include a racing mind, obsessive thoughts, unending worry, muscle tension and spasm, poor appetite or too great an appetite, digestive disorders, constipation, insomnia, poor blood flow, labored breathing, neck and shoulder tension, and the possible onset or continuation of bad habits such as dependence on alcohol, drugs, painkillers, food, and caffeine. Any one of these things by itself can trigger any number of different headaches. But when these forces of antagonism are combined (as they generally are when triggered by stress), the headache problem can become chronic and insufferable.

The sections that follow discuss the causes and effects of stress, the mind/body equation, and offer suggestions on how stress can be short-circuited and its headache triggers prevented from taking control of your body.

The Physiology of Stress

Stress is an interesting phenomenon; it means different things to different people. What we each individually consider to be stressful is largely a matter of our perception. Indeed, our perceptions are realities, and so what we think is posing a threat is actually doing so by virtue of our established belief system. Moreover, there are many kinds of stressors—physical (the response to being frightened), emotional (loss of a loved one), psychological (obsessive thoughts), spiritual (loss of faith), and psychosomatic (the need for attention).

From a physiological perspective, stress is responsible for initiating the fight-or-flight response in the face of perceived danger. This means that when we are confronted with a danger, our bodies automatically prepare us to deal with the coming stressful situation by focusing our attention, pumping more blood into our muscles to ready them for action, and by sending adrenaline through our systems. It is precisely this response that helps protect the body and return it again to homeostasis. However, too much stress or stress left unresolved for too long can lead to biological damage.

You see, at the onset of perceived danger the body is quickly jolted into fight-or-flight mode, which means stress hormones such as adrenaline and cortisol are pumped into the bloodstream. However, at the conclusion of the danger episode, the body does not as automatically calm down and return to homeostasis. In fact, it takes a great deal of time for the body to return to so-called normal conditions. But often this cannot happen because another stressor may present itself (e.g., sitting in traffic, standing in line at the bank, missing a deadline), and this will send our body into "code red" mode all over again.

The effects of such prolonged or recurring stress is that it keeps the autonomic nervous system from balancing, which can lead to problems with the gastrointestinal tract, digestive system, respiratory system, and neuroendocrine system and can lead to depression, anxiety, muscle tension, and insomnia. All of these are known triggers of tension-type headaches and migraine headaches.

Indeed, Zuzana Bic, Dr. P.H., and L. Francis Bic, Ph.D., warn that a number of the biochemical changes are induced by stress triggering the release of adrenaline, noradrenaline, and cortisol into the bloodstream, which increases levels of blood fat while decreasing levels of serotonin.[2]

The Mind/Body Connection

Headaches (and indeed illnesses in general) that have no definable biological cause yet do contain a mental/emotional/psychological component, are clinically termed psychosomatic. In the early days of this term's use a stigma was affixed to it that the health problems of its sufferers were "just in the mind" or "not real." But this couldn't be farther from the truth, for even though the related body symptom (in our case, headache pain) may have no underlying biological cause, the symptom is still felt in its very real manifestation by the one suffering it.

Perhaps a better term to use—and one that is central to the theme of this book—is mind/body. This is because psychosomatic illnesses are those which concurrently manifest both physical and mental components. "How could it be otherwise?" argues Andrew Weil, M.D. "Mind and body are two poles of our being, the nonphysical and the physical, which cannot exist apart from one another."[3]

Psychosomatic headaches, then, are those directly related to emotional disharmony and the stresses of life and our lifestyle choices, and they can be viewed as a cause-and-effect relationship. The headache pain is the direct effect of an unresolved emotional situation that manifests itself as stress, anxiety, and headache.

The Chinese character *yin/yang* represents this relationship well. It is a circle composed of two fishtail spheres: one black, the other white, and each containing color from the other. In pragmatic terms, this symbolizes the truth that there is no symptom without its underlying cause, just as there can be no light without dark and no sense of what is right without first identifying what is wrong. The cause-and-effect pattern in those who suffer chronic headaches is circular. Let's take a look at how this vicious circle of cause and effect can take hold in the body and transform vitality into illness.

If we are late for work and are stuck in traffic, the traffic jam and the passing time can be stressors. If we are breaking up with a significant other, the confrontation and unknown future can be stressors. If we are on a diet and sneak a piece of cake, the action of cheating can be a stressor.

Try to remember feelings you may have experienced when you were forced to do something you really did not want to do—either by someone else or through your own sense of obligation. For whatever moral, emotional, or psychological reason you did not want to perform this task—let's say, firing an employee or breaking up with a significant other—yet were pressured to do so in a timely manner. If you procrastinated or obsessed over it until the final moment, then afterwards did not express your negative emotions in an acceptable way but held them inside, the repressed anger, rage, resentment, frustration, and/or hatred manifested itself as stress and tension in the body, as muscle spasms and rise in blood pressure, as acid in the stomach, and eventually as headache.

Another example of the vicious cause-and-effect cycle is readily seen in our workforce, wherein productivity and the meeting of deadlines and bottom-line expectations lead us down a harrowing headache path. Consider the average day in the life of a corporate worker: Wakes up early, skips breakfast, and rushes to the office. Begins harboring stress and anxiety while watching the clock sitting in traffic. Once at work, sits all day at the computer and on the phone. Takes breaks not to stretch and breathe fresh air, but to artificially stimulate the body to work harder with cigarettes, sugar, and caffeine. Then back to work, pushing productivity in an attempt to meet expectations wherein stress and tensions rise and take hold of the body. After work, attempts to relax may include joining coworkers for happy hour, with intake of more caffeine, cigarettes, and alcohol. These habits go on day after day, until the body rebels and indicates something is very wrong by way of an ulcer, gastrointestinal disorder, or chronic headaches.

The mind/body (psychosomatic) headache can be described as the following chain reaction: Some external problem or dilemma not properly dealt with leads to stress, which manifests as muscle tension and spasm, leading to vertebral misalignment which is not only annoying, but leads to more tension in the body, irritated or pinched nerves (which cause referred head pain), and further stress. Further stress leads to liver damage, elevation of body heat and dehydration, insomnia, anxiety, a racing mind, and shortness of breath. Attempts to self-medicate these symptoms—taking analgesics and sleeping pills, consuming caffeine to stay awake in the morning, and turning to substances and comfort foods (such as wine, chocolate) to reduce the stress and anxiety—wreak further physiological havoc: Blood sugar levels rise, serotonin levels drop, and insulin is released in order to lower blood sugar, leading to a back-and-forth dilation and constriction of blood vessels, which induces rebound headaches.

Dr. Oliver Sacks has this to say about psychosomatic headaches: "The majority of patients who experience very frequent, severe, and unremitting migraines, for which no obvious circumstantial antecedents can be traced, are reacting to chronically difficult, intolerable, and even frightful life situations. In such patients we are able to observe or to infer powerful emotional stresses and needs . . . [driving] recurrent attacks."[4]

Just imagine, all of that from a so-called "make-believe" diagnosis of psychosomatic. From this, we can now see what Eastern healers have known all along: The mind and body, physical and emotional states are interconnected as intricately as the World Wide Web, and equally interdependent in terms of illness and healing.

Preventing Psychosomatic Headaches

This next section offers a number of examples of things you can do to better manage your existing psychosomatic or mind/body headaches, and prevent future ones from occurring. Since we have seen that these types of headaches have many causes and are linked to many symptoms, methods are presented for dealing with underlying psychological issues as well as physiological responses and mental centering.

WHEN PERCEPTION ISN'T REALITY

Stress headaches arise as a symptom (effect) of our innate physiological responses to "danger" situations. By this we mean any situation that has the ability to harm us now (e.g., a mugger) or later (e.g., a missed deadline at work). As mentioned earlier, this danger is rooted in our perception of its relevance to our life in some way. In these terms, the headache can be thought of as a physiological breakdown akin to a nervous breakdown in its effect of allowing us a socially acceptable "excuse" to rest or retreat from a situation.

As the doctors and researchers have shown us, our inability to deal with stress creates severe biochemical imbalances in our body and prevents it from reestablishing homeostasis. Remember that the overriding premise of the integrated mind/body headache prevention program is that if our body is at homeostasis there will be no headache. Therefore, without learning to come to terms with our perceptions that cause the stress that leads to physiological, psychological, physical, and emotional triggers that cause headaches, we can never truly become headache free.

The first step, then, is to realize that perceptions and realities do not always jibe. When we think something is life-threatening, as when a car suddenly pulls out in front of us, it may not actually be so. In addition, while we may think our boss will fire us if we are late with a report, this too may not be the case. What you need to do, then, is to develop a healthy outlook on the many components of your life and learn how you, personally and individually, can adjust to the stressful situations.

One way is to always do the best job you possibly can, whatever your vocation or hobby or relationship. Another is to always be honest with yourself regarding your talents, skills, and feelings and then by extension to be honest with those who depend on you. Try to set realistic goals and expectations in all aspects of your life, and keep those involved in these aspects abreast of things as they develop. For example, if you are stuck in traffic and will be late for a meeting, use a cell phone or pull over and make a simple phone call. This may cause you to be even later than if you stayed in traffic, but those awaiting your arrival will know where you are and expect the delay, thereby relieving the stress resulting from your perception of how they will react when you come in late. If your feelings are going astray in your relationship, talk to your partner before things get bad enough that the relationship disintegrates. Communication is also the best way of keeping anxieties and obsessions from getting the better of you and from causing insomnia, eating disorders, and other physiological responses to stress.

In short, you must learn to change your perceptions of what is threatening to you and just how threatening it really is. The examples offered are just a few and should help you in your personal journey toward dealing with everyday stressors. You may find in short time that those things which seemed to matter the most—and thus stress you the most—are really insignificant in the grand scheme of things.

CENTERING MIND AND EMOTIONS

Since the mind controls and constructs perceptions, and the emotions act and react toward threatening stimuli, the daily centering of mind and emotions is essential to headache prevention. While there are many methods of centering mind and emotions, I personally engage in daily meditation for at least 15 minutes—but often remain in the meditative state for up to 40 minutes or longer because it feels so good.

Meditation is practiced in as many ways as there are cultures in the world. Each country, each religion has its own means of meditation as spiritual discipline, healing practice, and/or mechanism for psychological growth. Regardless of method, practitioners continue to engage in meditation because they find it empowering, rewarding, healing, meaningful, peaceful . . . you name it. For chronic headache sufferers and those under constant stress and anxiety, it can be life-transforming.

In *Mosby's Complementary and Alternative Medicine*, authors L. W. Freeman and G. F. Lawlis include among a list of areas where meditation is successful as medical intervention, the following known headache triggers and symptoms: chronic pain, gastrointestinal distress, anxiety and panic, sleep disturbances, job and family stress, Type A behavior, and panic disorders.[5]

Moreover, in the section on "Meditation in Health Care Settings" in her exhaustive work, *Best Practices in Complementary and Alternative Med-*

icine, Dr. Lynda Freeman, Ph.D., states: "In clinical trials, mindfulness meditation has been demonstrated to effectively reduce anxiety and depression, including the condition known as post-traumatic stress; to significantly reduce chronic pain caused by a variety of medical conditions; to increase life functioning; and to reduce mood disturbances and psychiatric symptoms."[6]

The large-scale integration of meditation into medical settings happened in Boston, largely through the tireless efforts of Herbert Benson, M.D., and Jon Kabat-Zinn, Ph.D. After researching meditation techniques across many cultures, with a specific focus on the Transcendental Meditation of Maharishi Mahesh Yogi, Dr. Benson came to develop what is known simply as the Relaxation Response. This is a nonsecular method of inducing relaxation—that is, diminishing arousal of the sympathetic nervous system—by means of recitation of a single word and a passive attitude. Dr. Kabat-Zinn, on the other hand, was able to bring to the medical clinic the practice of Mindfulness Meditation—that is, the practice of being in the moment and not passing judgment on it while being aware of internal and external experience. Dr. Kabat-Zinn's program is called Mindfulness-Based Stress Reduction, or MBSR.

Both of these meditative/relaxation methods have proven clinically effective. In fact, an article by Dr. Kabat-Zinn reporting on a 1982 study and published in *General Hospital Psychiatry* stated: "65 percent of pain patients completing a MBSR Mindfulness Meditation program showed a reduction of greater than or equal to 33 percent in the mean total pain rating index, and 50 percent of patients showed a reduction greater than or equal to 50 percent. There were also significant . . . reductions in mood disturbances and psychiatric symptomatology."[7]

The meditation method I find most effective in my own personal management of stress, anxiety, insomnia, and headache is Vipassana or mindfulness meditation. While this meditative discipline comes from the Theravada sect of Buddhism as practiced in Southeast Asia, I do not practice Buddhism and neither must you to glean tremendous benefit from the method. In fact, the practice of mindfulness is secular and requires only dedication to yourself for a period of time each day.

Stress and anxiety generally prevent us from seeing or perceiving situations as they are because our minds begin to race with thoughts of what might happen "if" this or that happens or doesn't happen. Practitioners of mindfulness meditation liken this racing mind to a wild monkey. You must tame the wild monkey, they say, or it will forever be out of control. But by quieting the mind—that is, harnessing the racing thoughts and remaining calm and focused—your thoughts and emotions will be in your complete control when exasperating situations arise. This will then give you the ability to see situations clearly and be calm in emotion, focused in thought, and able to act rather than react to situations with full intention.

While it is not necessary, it is best for novices to find a quiet space and block of time in which they will not be disturbed. Wear loose-fitting clothing and be sure to relieve yourself beforehand. You should also not be too hungry nor too full, but comfortably satisfied and at ease. Limiting distractions is a must in order to reap any benefit from this practice. Here's how to do it:

1. Sit or lie down in any comfortable position that allows your spine to be straight and your head aligned with it.

2. Close your eyes and take a few initial deep breaths to ease into the moment and begin to relax.

3. Focus your attention on your breath as it passes into and out of the tip of your nose.

4. As you inhale, merely observe, without mental comment, the sensation you feel at the tip of your nose.

5. As you exhale, do the same thing.

6. If thoughts enter your mind, do not pass judgment on them. Merely acknowledge that they are there, allow them to pass, and return to the task of observing the sensation of the breath on the tip of the nose.

In the beginning stages you may have a tendency to fall asleep—or perhaps your mind may appear to race more than usual (it probably isn't racing, but your senses are closed and so you are just noticing your thoughts more fully). Your legs may fall asleep or tingle from poor flexibility or cramping. You may unknowingly lose focus of your breathing and find that your mind has wandered to another part of your body or to a drifting thought; this is okay.

Mindfulness meditation is about being *mindful* of your breath, your thoughts, the tension in your body, and so on. Continued practice will eradicate such obstructions, freeing your mind and spirit to act on more important things. However, this takes time. In the meantime, consider all of these distractions as a microcosm of your life. Every day you deal with multiple people talking with you at once, dozens of sounds flooding your ears, and disruptions in work. And as in this meditation, as these distractions arise you simply acknowledge them and then return to the task at hand, whether it's being mindful of your breathing or focused on your business pitch or deciding between two pressing circumstances when you really need to be doing a third.

There are many benefits to the daily practice of mindfulness meditation, including improved concentration, enhanced focus, unshakable emotions, inner fortitude, understanding of the self, objectivity, concentrated decision-making power, and peace of mind. Physiologically, you will experience a decrease in blood pressure, respiration, and metabolism, a calmer nervous system, hormone and chemical balance, and your body's return to its natural harmonious state of homeostasis.

Perhaps the most powerful effect of disciplined and prolonged meditative practice is the ability to live in the moment. That is, removing the past and future, knowing that there is only *now* and that every taste, smell, task, event, and thing you say or do now is all there is, and experiencing it to its fullest potential. So the next time you feel overwhelmed or anxious, take a moment to close your eyes, focus your mind, and breathe with mindful attention. Everything will fall into place when you open your eyes again.

Chapter Nine

A HEADACHE INTERVENTION
TECHNIQUE

Thus far we have come to understand headaches in terms of their many types and triggers. We have also come to understand the integrated mind/body approach to curing headache and how it works by preventing headache triggers from taking hold in the body. This approach to ridding headaches from our lives is based on a comprehensive modification in lifestyle choices. Since we are all humans, and therefore fallible, it is a given that we will at times fall off the wagon and indulge in things that may allow headaches back into our lives.

If you have reordered your life and reestablished homeostasis as directed, then your body will be more sensitive to the headache triggers than before. Therefore, if it took several drinks, cigarettes, and cups of coffee to trigger a headache prior to beginning this program, it may only take one glass of red wine to send you to bed in pain after you have been fully detoxed and rejuvenated. And so, that cappuccino with a double shot of espresso you will down "just this once" to get you through a damp December morning will instantly change your blood sugar, nerve functions, and respiration and affect the gastrointestinal tract, thus triggering a migraine. It will hurt, and you will want to take an analgesic "just this once" to get through it and carry on with your day.

My advice is this: Don't do it!

Not only will the caffeine in that cup of coffee throw your bodily systems off-kilter, but the analgesic will also affect your gastrointestinal tract, begin the process of toxic buildup again, and the combination of these two substances hold the promise of a rebound headache later in the day. If this happens, you're sure to take another analgesic, feel terrible, eat some chocolate, feel like you failed yourself, harbor stress in the muscles, take a drink after work out of self-pity, get another headache, and take another analgesic . . . and round and round you'll go until you are right back where you started with the return of chronic headaches.

While most headache books and programs offer a list of folk remedies for dealing with specific types of headache attacks (cluster, migraine, etc.), it is unrealistic to think you will be in the presence of mind to determine which type of headache you are having and then have the necessary herbs or aromatherapy oils on hand to do the trick.

If you fall off the wagon and a headache takes hold, I highly recommend you call in late for work—or leave early, depending on when the pain arises—and go through the following integrated mind/body intervention technique to greatly diminish or entirely remove the pain and allow you to return to your normal routine—without swallowing a painkiller. It is a simple sequence of things to do that, if done at the onset of the headache, will cancel out the triggers before they are able to truly take hold in the body and wreak havoc. It is a sequence that combines elements of the eight-part paradigm of headache prevention, but in a condensed and effective "quick fix" mode.

The technique sequence should bring lasting relief within 30 minutes to an hour. Here's the seven-part sequence:

✦ Drink three twelve-ounce bottles of spring water or purified water in one sitting. While you may find it difficult to do so, try your best to drink all three bottles within 5 to 10 minutes. This will help hydrate and detoxify the body.

✦ Breathe deeply and slowly while pressing and/or massaging the following acupressure points on the body: (1) the space between the big toe and second toe; (2) the webbing between the index finger and thumb; (3) the "third eye" or forehead location between the eyebrows; (4) the temples; (5) the earlobes; and (6) the base of the skull. This sequence will help reduce symptoms related to stress and organ functions.

✦ Submerge your hands or feet in very hot water, as hot as you can stand without burning yourself. This will draw blood away from the head and toward the hands, thereby reducing some of the vascular dilation and by extension the throbbing in the temporal arteries.

✦ Administer yourself a water enema as directed on the package. Evacuate your bowels and bladder.

✦ Take a temperature-therapy shower, preferably with no soap or shampoo. (They can be toxic.) Stand under the shower head and allow the water to pour directly over your head and shoulders. Begin with very hot water, and after 5 or more minutes change it to cold water for a time. Return again to hot water and then reduce the water to body temperature, which is the temperature where you can barely feel the water because it matches the temperature of your own body. The combination of the hot-water hand soak and this hot/cold/hot/body temperature shower will stabilize the blood vessels, which may have been constricting and dilating.

✦ Put on loose-fitting clothes that will not obstruct breathing, lie down, and engage in cyclical breathing (4 counts in and 8 counts out) followed by progressive relaxation or mindfulness meditation, as you feel is needed.

✦ Drifting off to sleep for even 10 minutes will also help, especially if the headache was in part brought on by sleep deprivation or stress.

This sequence takes between 30 minutes and 1 hour to complete, but it is necessary to perform all measures in an effort to abort the single-type or mixed headache in progress before it has had a chance to really take hold in your body. It will work if you allow it to work, by relaxing and letting each part do its job. If you are worried about getting someplace fast or try to force the technique, it will only add stress, anxiety, labored breathing, irritation, and confound the headache onset in progress. However, if you follow the sequence and give yourself the time necessary to complete it, you will not further aggravate the situation or reintroduce toxins into your system, and you will be able to get on with the day with much less of a headache, or none at all.

Afterword

We have come to a point in our society and lives where it is evident that we cannot expect others to do for us what we must do for ourselves. While advances in surgical procedures are astounding, and while we are living longer than at any other time in history, we are also suffering greatly along the way. It should be evident by now that where non-biologically induced headaches are concerned, we are personally the cause of our chronic suffering. And it is precisely because we are the cause of our condition that it is only we who can rid the headaches from our own lives. In other words, we can be both cause and cure, and it is our choice which we one choose to be.

If you choose to be your own best friend and not your most feared foe, you must embrace the integrated mind/body headache prevention approach explained and taught in this book. And the success of this approach to curing headaches is absolutely rooted in the positive modification of your lifestyle and worldview. Without changing how you perceive the world around you, and the cause of your pain and suffering, then you will never live headache free—ever. The pain will keep recurring, over and over, and the more medicine you take to deaden the pain, the more you will exacerbate the condition and the worse and more damaging it will become.

I urge you to read this book through several times over the next few weeks. Come to understand why and how the program works so that you will believe in it. If you can believe in the program's abilities and you can believe in your own willingness and stamina to follow it through, it will become habit and your lifestyle will change as necessary without psychologically painful effort. I want you to follow this program because I traveled the world in search of a cure and developed one based on the methods and research of physicians and healers and my own personal experience as a severe headache sufferer for almost thirty dreadful years. I want you to be pain-free, too, and I know it will happen if you dedicate to yourself the necessary time, energy, and love. I wish you much success and happiness for the rest of your healthy and headache-free life.

References Cited

Chapter 1

1. Mayo Clinic, "Migraines: Taking Control of Your Pain." *Mayo Clinic Women's Health Source* (August 1997).

2. Jackie Sieppert, "Attitudes Toward and Knowledge of Chronic Pain: A Survey of Medical Social Workers." *Health & Social Work* (May 1996).

3. The American Occupational Therapy Association, "Managing Chronic Pain." www.aota.org (December 2002).

4. OnHealth.com, "Chronic Pain: Causes and Treatments. " (July 1999).

5. ABCNEWS.com, "Health & Living." (December 4, 1998).

6. Landmark Health Care, Inc, "Report 1: On Public Perception of Alternative Care." www.landmarkhealthcare.com/LMReport1.html (1998).

7. Landmark Health Care, Inc., "Report II: On HMOs and Alternative Care." www.landmarkhealthcare.com/LMReport11.html (1999).

8. David Eisenberg and Roger B. Davis, et al, "Trends in Alternative Medicine Use in the United States, 1990–1997." *Journal of the American Medical Association* 280 (1998): 1569–1575.

9. John A. Astin, "Why Patients Use Alternative Medicine." *Journal of the American Medical Association: Results of a National Study* 279 (1998): 1548–1553.

10. Zuzana Bic, G. C. Blix, et al, "In Search of the Ideal Treatment for Migraine Headache." *Medical Hypothesis* 50 (January 1998): 1–7.

11. Zuzana Bic, G. C. Blix, et al, "The Influence of a Low-Fat Diet on Incidence and Severity of Migraine Headaches." *Journal of Women's Health & Gender-Based Medicine* 8, no. 5 (June 1999): 5.

12. Zuzana Bic and L. Francis Bic, *No More Headaches, No More Migraines* (Garden City, NY: Avery Publishing Group, 1999), 2.

13. R. Milne, B. More, et al, *Definitive Guide to Headaches* (Tiburon, CA: Future Medicine Publishing, 1997), 56.

14. Ruth A. Mack, "The Art of Striking Back." *The D.O.* (July 1991), 88.

Chapter 2

1. R. Milne, B. More, et al, *Definitive Guide to Headaches* (Tiburon, CA: Future Medicine Publishing, 1997), 56.

2. Ibid.

3. Zuzana Bic and L. Francis Bic, *No More Headaches, No More Migraines* (Garden City, NY: Avery Publishing Group, 1999).

4. R. Milne, B. More, et al, *Definitive Guide to Headaches* (Tiburon, CA: Future Medicine Publishing, 1997), 60.

5. R. Milne, B. More, et al, *Definitive Guide to Headaches* (Tiburon, CA: Future Medicine Publishing, 1997), 57.

6. Oliver Sacks, *Migraine* (New York: Vintage Books, 1992), 213.

7. Bob Flaws, *Migraines and Traditional Chinese Medicine: A Layperson's Guide* (Boulder, CO: Blue Poppy Press, 1990).

Chapter 3

1. Zuzana Bic and L. Francis Bic, *No More Headaches, No More Migraines* (Garden City, NY: Avery Publishing Group, 1999), 73.

2. Stagliano, *The D.O.* (July 1991), 86.

3. Andrew Weil, *Health and Healing* (Boston: Houghton Mifflin, 1988), 62.

4. Daniel Reed, *Chi-Kung: Harnessing the Power of the Universe* (Great Britain: Simon and Schuster, 1998), 107.

5. Vijayendra Pratap, *Beginning Yoga* (Boston: Tuttle Publishing, 1997), 85–89.

6. FaXiang Hou and Mark V. Wiley, *Qigong for Health and Well-Being* (Boston: Journey Editions, 1998).

Chapter 4

1. Alma E. Guinness, ed., *The ABC's of the Human Body* (New York: The Reader's Digest Association, 1987), 262.

2. F. Batmanghelidj, *Your Body's Many Cries for Water* (Falls Church, VA: Global Health Solutions, 1996), 11.

3. www.PhenomeNEWS.com. "An exclusive interview with Dr. Batmanghelidj." www.phenomenews.com/archives/may01/batman .html, 2001.

4. R. Milne, B. More, et al, *Definitive Guide to Headaches* (Tiburon, CA: Future Medicine Publishing, 1997), 112–13.

5. United States Environmental Protection Agency, "819 Cities Exceed Lead Levels for Drinking Water," Environmental Protection Agency Environmental News, Publication #A-107 (May 11, 1993), p. 110.

6. United States Environmental Protection Agency, "How Safe is My Drinking Water?" www.epa.gov/safewater/wrot/howsafe.html.

7. R. Milne, B. More, et al, *Definitive Guide to Headaches* (Tiburon, CA: Future Medicine Publishing, 1997), 11.

8. Rudolph Ballentine, *Radical Healing* (New York: Harmony Books, 1999), 290.

9. www.PhenomeNEWS.com. "An exclusive interview with Dr. Batmanghelidj." www.phenomenews.com/archives/may01/batman.html, 2001.

Chapter 5

1. Gallo, Anthony E. "Food Advertising in the United States." www.ers.usda.gov/publications/aib750/aib750i.pdf (1997), 175.

2. Elson M. Haas, *The Detox Diet* (Berkeley, CA: Celestial Arts, 1996), 22.

3. Oliver Sacks, *Migraine* (New York: Vintage Books, 1992), 155.

4. D. Y. Graham, et al, "The Effects of Bran on Bowel Function in Constipation." *American Journal of Gastroenterology* 77 (1982): 599–603.

5. Rudolph Ballentine, *Radical Healing.* (New York: Harmony Books, 1999), 288.

6. Elson M. Haas, *The Detox Diet* (Berkeley, CA: Celestial Arts, 1996), 7.

7. Paavo Airola, *How to Get Well* (Phoenix, AZ: Health Plus Publishers, 1974), 123.

8. Elson M. Haas, *The Detox Diet* (Berkeley, CA: Celestial Arts, 1996), 107.

Chapter 6

1. Ted Broer, *Maximum Energy* (Lake Mary, FL: Ailoam Press, 1999), 65.

2. Health Square.com. "Why We Get Headaches." Excerpted from Chapter 14 of *The PDR Family Guide to Women's Health* (Montvale, NJ: Thomson Healthcare, 1994).

3. Ted Broer, *Maximum Energy* (Lake Mary, FL: Ailoam Press, 1999), 57–58.

Chapter 7

1. Shery Brourman, *Walk Yourself Well* (New York: Hyperion, 1996).

2. Josh Holzer, *Warrior Walking* (Burbank, CA: Multi-Media Books, 1999).

3. Wang Xuanjie and J. P. C. Moffett, *Traditional Chinese Therapeutic Exercises—Standing Pole* (Beijing, China: Foreign Language Press, 1994), 40.

4. China Sports Editorial Board. *Liangong in 18 Exercises* (Hong Kong: Hai Feng Publishing Co., 1992).

5. R. Milne and B. More, et al, *Definitive Guide to Headaches* (Tiburon, CA: Future Medicine Publishing, 1997), 118.

Chapter 8

1. Oliver Sacks, *Migraine* (New York: Vintage Books, 1992).

2. Zuzana Bic and L. Francis Bic, *No More Headaches, No More Migraines* (Garden City, NY: Avery Publishing Group, 1999), 91.

3. Andrew Weil, *Health and Healing* (Boston: Houghton Mifflin, 1988), 57.

4. Oliver Sacks, *Migraine* (New York: Vintage Books, 1992), 172.

5. L. W. Freeman and G. F. Lawlis, *Mosby's Complementary and Alternative Medicine: A Research-based Approach* (St. Louis, MO: Mosby, 2001).

6. Lynda Freeman, *Best Practices in Complementary and Alternative Medicine: An Evidence-Based Approach with Nursing CE/CME* (Gaithersburg, MD: Aspen Publications, 2001).

7. Jon Kabat-Zinn, "An Outpatient Program in Behavioral Medicine for Chronic Pain Patients Based on the Practice of Mindfulness Meditation: Theoretical Considerations and Preliminary Results." *General Hospital Psychiatry* 4, no. 1 (1982): 33–47.

Bibliography

ABCNEWS.com. "Health & Living." (December 4,1998).

Airola, Paavo. *How to Get Well*. Phoenix, AZ: Health Plus Publishers, 1974.

Astin, John A. "Why Patients Use Alternative Medicine." *Journal of the American Medical Association: Results of a National Study* 279 (1998): 1548–1553.

Ballentine, Rudolph. *Radical Healing*. New York: Harmony Books, 1999.

Batmanghelidj, F. *Your Body's Many Cries for Water*. Falls Church, VA: Global Health Solutions, 1996.

Benson, Herbert. *The Relaxation Response*. New York: Avon Books, 1975.

Bhikkhu, Buddhadasa. *Mindfulness with Breathing*. Boston: Wisdom Publications, 1996.

Bic, Zuzana and L. Francis Bic. *No More Headaches, No More Migraines*. Garden City, NY: Avery, 1999.

Bic, Zuzana, G. C. Blix, et al. "In Search of the Ideal Treatment for Migraine Headache." *Medical Hypothesis* 50 (January 1998).

Bic, Zuzana, G. C. Blix, et al. "The Influence of a Low-Fat Diet on Incidence and Severity of Migraine Headaches." *Journal of Women's Health & Gender-Based Medicine* 8, no. 5. (June 1999).

Broer, Ted. *Maximum Energy*. Lake Mary, FL: Ailoam Press, 1999.

Brourman, Shery. *Walk Yourself Well*. New York: Hyperion, 1996.

Burks, Susan L. *Managing Your Migraine: A Migraine Sufferer's Practical Guide.* Totowa, NJ: Humana Press, 1994.

China Sports Editorial Board. *Liangong in 18 Exercises.* Hong Kong: Hai Feng Publishing Co., 1992.

Delvecchio Good, M., Bradwin, P. et al. *Pain as Human Experience: An Anthropological Perspective.* Berkeley, CA: University of California Press, 1992.

Donsbach, Kurt, W. *Vitamins and Minerals Revised.* Huntington Beach, CA: The International Institute of Natural Health Sciences, 1981.

Eisenberg, David. *Encounters with Qi: Exploring Chinese Medicine.* New York: W.W. Norton and Company, 1995.

Eisenberg, David and Roger B. Davis, et al. "Trends in Alternative Medicine Use in the United States, 1990–1997." *Journal of the American Medical Association* 280 (1998): 1569–1575.

Flaws, Bob. *Migraines and Traditional Chinese Medicine: A Layperson's Guide.* Boulder, CO: Blue Poppy Press, 1990.

Freeman, L. W. & Lawlis, G. F. *Mosby's Complementary and Alternative Medicine: A Research-based Approach.* St. Louis, MO: Mosby, 2001.

Freeman, Lynda. *Best Practices in Complementary and Alternative Medicine: An Evidence-Based Approach with Nursing CE/CME.* Gaithersburg, MD: Aspen Publications, 2001.

Goleman, Daniel. *The Meditative Mind.* Los Angeles: Jeremy P. Tarcher, Inc., 1988.

Graham, D. Y. et al. "The Effects of Bran on Bowel Function in Constipation." *American Journal of Gastroenterology* 77 (1982): 599–603.

Guinness, Alma E., ed. *The ABC's of the Human Body.* New York: The Reader's Digest Association, 1987.

Gunaratana, Henepola. *Mindfulness in Plain English.* Boston: Wisdom Publications, 1991.

Haas, Elson M. *The Detox Diet*. Berkeley, CA: Celestial Arts, 1996.

Harris, Gail. *Body and Soul*. New York: Kensington Books, 1999.

Hoffman, Ronald. *Intelligent Medicine*. New York: Fireside Books, 1997.

Holzer, Josh. *Warrior Walking: A Guide to Walking as Exercise, Meditation and Self-Defense*. Burbank, CA: Multi-Media Books, 1999.

Hou, FaXiang & Mark V. Wiley. *Qigong for Health and Well-Being*. Boston: Journey Editions, 1998.

Kabat-Zinn, Jon. "An Outpatient Program in Behavioral Medicine for Chronic Pain Patients Based on the Practice of Mindfulness Meditation: Theoretical Considerations and Preliminary Results." *General Hospital Psychiatry* 4, no. 1 (1982).

Landmark Health Care, Inc. "Report 1: On Public Perception of Alternative Care." www.landmarkhealthcare.com/LMReport1.html (1998).

Landmark Health Care, Inc. "Report II: On HMOs and Alternative Care." www.landmarkhealthcare.com/LMReport11.html (1999).

Mack, Ruth A. "The Art of Striking Back." *The D.O.* (July 1991).

Mayo Clinic. "Migraines: Taking Control of Your Pain." *Mayo Clinic Women's Health Source*. (August 1997).

Milne, R., B. More, et al. *Definitive Guide to Headaches*. Tiburon, CA: Future Medicine Publishing, 1997.

OnHealth.com. "Chronic Pain: Causes and Treatments." (July 1999).

PhenomeNEWS.com. "An Exclusive Interview with Dr. Batmanghelidj." www.phenomenews.com/archives/may01/batman.html (2001).

Philips, H. C. and S. Rachman. *The Psychological Management of Chronic Pain*. New York: Springer Publishing Co., 1996.

Pratap, Vijayendra. *Beginning Yoga*. Boston: Tuttle Publishing, 1997.

Reed, Daniel. *Chi-Kung: Harnessing the Power of the Universe*. Great Britain: Simon and Schuster, 1998.

Sacks, Oliver. *Migraine.* New York: Vintage Books, 1992.

Sieppert, Jackie. "Attitudes Toward and Knowledge of Chronic Pain: A Survey of Medical Social Workers." *Health & Social Work.* (May 1996).

Stagliano. *The D.O.* (July 1991).

American Occupational Therapy Association, Inc. "Managing Chronic Pain." www.aota.org (December 2002).

United States Environmental Protection Agency. "819 Cities Exceed Lead Levels for Drinking Water," *Environmental Protection Agency Environmental News, Publication #A-107* (May 11, 1993).

United States Environmental Protection Agency. "How Safe is My Drinking Water?" www.epa.gov/safewater/wrot/howsafe.html.

Xuanjie Wang and J. P. C. Moffett. *Traditional Chinese Therapeutic Exercises—Standing Pole.* Beijing, China: Foreign Language Press, 1994.

Weil, Andrew. *Health and Healing.* Boston: Houghton Mifflin, 1988.

About the Author

A survivor of nearly thirty years of incapacitating headaches, Mark V. Wiley, OMD., traveled the world in search of a cure and developed one based on in-depth research and his personal experiences at the hands of physicians, psychologists, chiropractors, acupuncturists, bone setters, faith healers, and shamans. A doctor of Oriental medicine, practitioner of acupuncture, and master of qigong and tuina, Dr. Wiley is a medical writer for HealUSA.net and former publisher of *Quality of Life* and 247You.com, as well as product development manager for Agora Health. He lectures and gives seminars internationally on qigong and martial arts. He is the author of nine books on health, martial arts, and Asian culture, and his articles have appeared in magazines and journals worldwide. He lives in Philadelphia, where he practices integrated energy medicine.

OTHER OUTWITTING TITLES YOU MAY ENJOY

Outwitting Back Pain *(coming in Fall 2004)*

Outwitting Housework

Outwitting Insomnia

Outwitting the Job Market

Outwitting Stress

Outwitting Writer's Block